AS FEATURED BY JEAN CARPER IN *USA WEEKEND*

"Finally, a book by a renowned and active researcher that proves the value of nutritional supplements. *The Antioxidant Miracle* provides a shield protecting us from disease and ensuring health. **The information in this book could save your life!**"

> —Julian Whitaker, M.D., founder, Whitaker Wellness Institute
> and editor, *Health and Healing*

"One of the world's leading authorities on antioxidants."

> —Jean Carper, author of *Miracle Cures* and *Stop Aging Now!* in *USA Weekend*

"*The Antioxidant Miracle* is **informative, timely, and well written**. I have treated patients with therapeutic doses of antioxidant supplements for over 20 years and have seen astounding results."

> —Burt Berkson, M.D., coauthor of *Syndrome X: The Complete*
> *Nutritional Program to Prevent and Reverse Insulin Resistance*

"Life is like a candle flame, and antioxidants make it burn brighter and longer. Lester Packer is the keeper of the flame. For those of us seeking to combat the debility and diseases of aging, *The Antioxidant Miracle* is **an essential tool.**"

> —William Regelson, M.D., coauthor of *The Melatonin Miracle*

"Any health-conscious person will want to read *The Antioxidant Miracle.* It makes the understanding of these miracle nutrients **easy to comprehend and utilize** in his or her everyday life."

> —Earl Mindell, Ph.D., author of *The Herb Bible* and *The Vitamin Bible*

"Antioxidants are the key to twenty-first century medicine. Dr. Lester Packer and Carol Colman explain the importance of these wondrous micronutrients—and which ones to take and why. I could not practice medicine without antioxidants, especially lipoic acid. **Read *The Antioxidant Miracle* and find out why you should never be without your dose of lipoic acid.**"

> —Fred Pescatore, M.D., author of *Thin For Good* and *Feed Your Kids Well*

The Antioxidant Miracle

Put Lipoic Acid, Pycnogenol, and Vitamins E and C to Work for You

Lester Packer, Ph.D.,
and Carol Colman

John Wiley & Sons, Inc.

New York • Chichester • Weinheim • Brisbane • Singapore • Toronto

To Michael, Anna, David, and Anne

Published by John Wiley & Sons, Inc.
Published simultaneously in Canada

Design and production by Navta Associates, Inc.

Originally published in hardcover as *The Antioxidant Miracle: Your Complete Plan for Total Health and Healing*

This publication is designed to provide accurate and authoritative information in regard to the subject matter covered. It is sold with the understanding that the publisher is not engaged in rendering professional services. If professional advice or other expert assistance is required, the services of a competent professional person should be sought. Pregnant women should not take supplements unless under a doctor's supervision.

Library of Congress Cataloging-in-Publication Data:
Packer, Lester.
    The antioxidant miracle : put lipoic acid, pycnogenol, and vitamins E and C to work for you / Lester Packer and Carol Colman.
        p.   cm.
    "Published simultaneously in Canada."
    Includes bibliographical references and index.
    ISBN 978-1-62045-619-4
    1. Antioxidants—Health aspects.   2. Thioctic acid—Health aspects.
3. Vitamin C—Health aspects.   4. Vitamin E—Health aspects.   5. Ubiquinones—Health aspects.   I. Colman, Carol.   II. Title.

RM666. A555 P33   2000
613.2'8—dc21   99-052442

Contents

Foreword

When Dr. Lester Packer asked me to write the foreword to *The Antioxidant Miracle*, I was delighted. Les Packer is the person who can make antioxidant science clear to the reader, for he has devoted his long and productive career to studying how antioxidants affect biological systems and how they might be able to extend the length and quality of human life.

Les and I first met in 1969 when I was on sabbatical leave at the University of California at Berkeley (where I had received my Ph.D.), spending six months on a Guggenheim Fellowship in the laboratory of Nobel laureate Melvin Calvin. Les approached me when I first arrived and said: "Let's teach a course on antioxidants and aging!" And we did!! That, so like Les, was the push that got me started teaching about free radical biology.

As it turned out, the year I arrived was an important one for the Packer Laboratory, with many experiments going on to solve the mystery of how oxygen (which is necessary for life) can also harm cells and how vitamin E and other antioxidants can be protective and extend cell life. That exciting year was my introduction to the field of free radical biology, a field in which Les was already an expert. Les brings insight and long experience to the biological side of the field, whereas I, with Les's help, was the first free radical chemist to turn to the full-time study of the effects of free radicals in biological systems.

Les and I have worked together on many projects over the years. In 1976, Les and I organized a Gordon Research Conference entitled "Oxygen Radicals in Biology." The Gordon Conferences bring together the best people in a research area and encourage them to talk openly (no recordings or quotations are permitted) about the ongoing research in their labs. Les had chaired Gordon Conference sections on energy coupling mechanisms, and in 1972 I had organized the first Gordon Conference on free radical chemistry, a conference that attempted to mix people interested in the chemistry and biological effects of radicals, to the happy advantage of each group. However, the

Gordon Conference on free radicals had been taken over by chemists, to the detriment of the biological side, so Les and I organized one that exclusively focused on the health effects of radicals and antioxidants.

I had written the first college textbook on free radicals (*Free Radicals,* 1966), but I knew very little about biology, so my 1969 sojourn at Berkeley with Les and Melvin Calvin's group was my introduction to free radical biology. Following that, free radical biology became my central interest. I later edited *Free Radicals in Biology and Medicine* (1972–1977), a six-volume set, and am currently coeditor in chief of the journal *Free Radical Biology & Medicine,* the premier journal in the field.

So, in short, Les and I became fast and lifelong friends from our first meeting in 1969. We are kindred spirits and share an intuition that understanding the interaction between antioxidants and free radicals—both at a chemical and biology level—could be the key to the tantalizing possibility of extending the healthy years for humans.

In the years since Les and I first began collaborating, antioxidants have become a burgeoning field of research that attracts the best and brightest scientists from all over the world. When Les and I started in the field, antioxidants were described only in the most elite and erudite scientific journals—and now every educated layperson is also knowledgeable and curious about radicals and antioxidants.

While nonscientists are aware of the importance of radicals and antioxidants in health, they are not always clear on just what the facts are. Clearly, we now stand at the threshold of a new understanding of how antioxidants can affect the quality and length of human life. Antioxidants in many systems can protect us against heart attacks, cancer, neurological diseases (including Alzheimer's), and other degenerative diseases of aging.

That these advances have occurred is in no small measure because of Lester Packer, who has been a major player and driving force in free radical biology for forty years. His remarkable energy and his prolific publications have resulted in groundbreaking research. Les is almost single-handedly responsible for a huge number of interdisciplinary exchanges through hundreds of international scientific meetings that he has organized.

The tradition of cross-fertilization, sharing of information, and close cooperation among scientists in different disciplines that has characterized the field of antioxidant research in the twenty years since the first Gordon Conference continues today. Recently, in my laboratory, we developed a new method of analyzing the free radicals in cigarette smoke and smoggy urban air, and we have studied the ways in which antioxidants can protect against these oxidative stresses. We also have been interested in the role of nitric oxide in the formation of chemically induced tumors (chemical carcinogenesis).

Les's group had been studying the role of nitric oxide in cells and is already conducting clinical trials to determine the efficacy of antioxidant cocktails in protecting both active and passive smokers from lung cancer. So once again, Les's and my research efforts have dovetailed.

You have in your hand a guidebook, written by a prominent scientist in the field, that can lead you into the wonderful world of antioxidants and human health. In this book, Les explains in simple, direct terms how you can best protect yourself against aging and degenerative diseases by taking formulations containing the key elements of the antioxidant network. His conclusions are based on research conducted in his laboratory at the University of California at Berkeley and at other important research centers throughout the world.

The fact that Lester Packer remains at the forefront of the intellectual and organizational leadership of his field long past retirement age makes him the living proof that antioxidant supplementation is a key to a longer, healthier life.

—William A. Pryor
Thomas & David Boyd Professor
Director of the Biodynamics Institute
Louisiana State University
Baton Rouge, La.

Acknowledgments

It is a pleasure to acknowledge those who helped to bring *The Antioxidant Miracle* into being.

I owe allegiance to the many students who, over the past three decades, have listened to my lectures in the physiology of aging course at the University of California at Berkeley and to colleagues in the scientific audiences that I have addressed who, through the years, have asked insightful questions about the importance of natural antioxidants that gave rise to this book.

It's marvelous when "necessity coincides with desire." Writing this book has been a valuable and rewarding experience because of my talented coauthor Carol Colman. Working together, we brought each other energy to get done what was needed at the right time to complete this project.

From the outset, Tom Miller, our editor, was very supportive and encouraging. His advice and wisdom helped to bring the book into focus. Tom's counsel was much appreciated. Also many thanks to our agent, Richard Curtis.

In a career that has spanned more than four decades, I've met many people who have been generous with their time, knowledge, and wisdom. I would like to thank some of them here. I owe a special debt of gratitude to Al Schatz, Morris Shils, and Carlton R. Bovell of Brooklyn College, my early mentors, who were responsible for igniting my lifelong interest in research. Through them I met Seymour Hutner and Luigi Provasoli of Haskins Laboratories, where I spent several fruitful years while I was a student.

Many thanks to the wonderful scientists I worked with at the University of Pennsylvania early in my career, including Britton Chance, Ronald W. Estabrook, and Martin Klingenberg, who have remained lifelong friends.

I would also like to thank some of my senior colleagues: David E. Green and Albert Lehninger for inspiration, and especially David Green, with whom I cofounded the U.S. Bioenergetics Group. This group, which is still flourishing, was the first interest group of the Biophysical

Society and became a model for other societies both nationally and internationally. When I was a chair at the Gordon Conferences of Energy Coupling Mechanisms, I had the privilege to work with and learn from David E. Green, Albert Lehninger, Paul Boyer, Britton Chance, and Peter Mitchell.

Many thanks to the University of London and Dennis Chapman in biomembrane and lipid research. In his lab at the Royal Free Hospital, I met Anthony Diplock of vitamin E fame and Catherine Rice-Evans of flavonoids and polyphenol fame in the early days of antioxidant research. Tony, Catherine, and I remain colleagues and close friends.

A very special thanks to my colleagues at the Packer Laboratory, including two very talented people, Valerian Kagan and Elena Serbinova, whose work has focused on the antioxidant network. The role of Coenzyme Q10 in the network was aided by the experiments of John Maguire, one of my longtime associates and friends. Many brilliant and devoted students and scholars have continued with these studies.

I am indebted to William Regelson for his encouragement to write a general book on antioxidants rather than to concentrate on one or two favorite antioxidants.

My endeavors in antioxidant research have also been nurtured by many visiting scholars, in particular, Akitane Mori and Helmet Sies, distinguished visiting professors who regularly visit the Packer Lab, and Bill Pryor, who through the years has been both a friend and a respected colleague. I would also like to acknowledge Dr. Arthur Furst, a famous toxicologist who is a brilliant, articulate scientist and a great role model.

I am especially grateful for the advice of several of my colleagues who read the text, in particular, Anne Packer, Sashwati Roy, and Arianna Carughi. Many thanks to Maret G. Traber, a wonderful friend and colleague who is one of the world's leading researchers on vitamin E. Her comments and suggestions were invaluable. I would also like to thank Sai Rangsit and Chris Berry for their inspiration and moral support, and Andrew Waterhouse, John Weisberger, and Norman Krinsky for their assistance. The critical insight and imagination offered by these friends and colleagues played an important role in shaping *The Antioxidant Miracle* into the book that I have endeavored to develop for the general public and the community of health professionals.

—Lester Packer, Ph.D.

Introduction

I believe in miracles, not in spite of the fact that I am a scientist, but *because* I am a scientist. All one has to do is consider the extraordinary scientific advances that have occurred in just the last half century, and one can't help but believe in miracles. I witness miracles in my laboratory and in the labs of my colleagues every day.

I am a professor and a member of the Department of Molecular and Cell Biology at the University of California at Berkeley, where I head the Packer Laboratory, one of the world's leading antioxidant research centers. Antioxidants are vitamins and minerals that are found in foods and also manufactured by our bodies. They are critical for optimal health. The Packer Lab is home to dozens of highly trained, brilliant scientists from around the world. Each day they learn something that will have a profound effect on our health and well-being.

The Antioxidant Miracle is the culmination of the nearly five decades of research that I have devoted to the study of antioxidants. It is my way of sharing with you the miracles we have witnessed at the Packer Lab. Literally thousands of studies have confirmed that antioxidants can help prevent numerous diseases and will not only enhance life, but in all probability extend life. It is my hope that this information will help readers live longer, healthier lives.

My interest in science—and in biology, particularly—began in more humble surroundings. I grew up in the Bronx. Even if you're not from New York, you know that the Bronx is about as urban an environment as they come, but even if you are from New York, you may not know that the borough's Van Courtland Park was an oasis of lakes and swamps full of amphibian species and bird life. One of my boyhood friends introduced me to the study of these creatures and together we joined the Dewitt Clinton High School Nature Study Club. By age sixteen, I was fairly proficient in the identification of bird species and became the youngest member of the Linnaean Society of New York of the American Museum of Natural History.

At Brooklyn College, my courses in microbiology were taught by Professor Albert Schatz, who discovered the antibiotic streptomycin when he was a graduate student. At his suggestion, I took a research course with him and assisted him in the laboratory. One of the most important lessons I learned from Al was that science must be practiced with meticulous precision. I would often help Al by washing the lab glassware—I would scrub each test tube and vial until it gleamed. Every day, Al would hold the glassware up to the light and scrutinize my work. If he could detect even a brush mark on the glassware, I would have to rewash it!

While I was still a student at Brooklyn College, Al introduced me to Seymore Hutner, who headed the Haskins Laboratories in New York, and he hired me as a research assistant. At the Haskins Laboratories I met Dr. Wolf Vishniac, a distinguished microbiologist who had returned from several years of postdoctoral training in the lab of C. B. VanNiel in Holland, who is revered as the father of microbiology. Dr. Vishniac had been recruited by Brooklyn College to teach a graduate course in microbiology, and I was honored when he asked me to be his laboratory assistant. It proved to be a huge challenge. I had to work around the clock, many nights catching only an hour or two of sleep in the laboratory before the students would arrive in the morning. Working on a tight budget, we were unable to buy all of the materials that Wolf required. In fact, I remember on my way to school keeping my eye out for any empty whiskey bottles I would find in the trash that could be used as storage containers. Whatever the school lacked in resources, Wolf more than made up for them with his enthusiasm and exceptional teaching technique. The course was enormously popular with the students, and a wonderful learning experience for me.

Wolf was invited to become an assistant professor in the Department of Microbiology at Yale, where I worked as his research assistant. In 1956, I earned my Ph.D. in microbiology and biochemistry, and then I went for postdoctoral studies with Britton Chance at the Johnson Research Foundation of the University of Pennsylvania School of Medicine. After a brief stint at the University of Texas, I joined the faculty of the University of California at Berkeley, home of the Packer Lab. Since then, much of my work has centered on two important antioxidants—vitamin E and a newly discovered antioxidant, lipoic acid.

For the past three decades, the Packer Lab has been the site of numerous breakthroughs in biology, which I will describe in *The Antioxidant Miracle*. You will learn about some startling new discoveries on the role of antioxidants and free radicals in the prevention and treatment of many chronic and degenerative diseases—including heart disease, cancer, arthritis, and cataracts.

In Part Four, The Packer Plan—Making the Antioxidant Miracle Work for You, I will outline the Packer Plan, my state-of-the-art antioxidant supplement, diet, and skin-care regimen.

Although I have written hundreds of scientific articles and dozens of scientific books, this is my first book for nonscientists. It gives me great pleasure to be able to share this vital, lifesaving information with the public.

PART ONE

The Antioxidant Advantage

1

The Antioxidant Miracle

Suppose that I told you there was a pill that would keep your heart strong, your mind sharp, and your body youthful well into your seventies, eighties, nineties, and even beyond? Suppose that I told you there was a pill that could extend your life and improve your sex life? Suppose I told you there was a pill that could prevent cancer? How about a pill that could keep your skin supple and wrinkle-free?

Would you think that I was a victim of wishful thinking? A weird futurist dreaming about a drug yet to be discovered? I'm not. I am a serious mainstream scientist, and the pills I am talking about not only really exist but are readily available. They are in your neighborhood pharmacy and natural food store. Chances are you will find them on the shelves of your local grocery and discount store. You can purchase them by phone, by mail, and by e-mail on the Internet. (You may have a few on your kitchen counter already—but you're probably not taking them correctly.) But their availability doesn't make their effects any less miraculous.

I am talking about antioxidants, a family of vitamins, minerals, and other nutrients that I have been studying for the better part of my seventy years. Antioxidants are the reason I get up every morning and go to my lab at the University of California at Berkeley. Antioxidants are the reason I travel all over the world to attend scientific conferences. Antioxidants are the reason I have written hundreds of scientific articles and, now, this book. And antioxidants are the reason why, at my age, I have no plans whatsoever to slow down. My name has become so closely linked to the study of antioxidants that I have been dubbed "Dr. Antioxidant" by some of my colleagues.

Antioxidants are a group of compounds that are produced by the body and that occur naturally in many foods. Antioxidants work together in the body to maintain our health and vigor well into the late decades of life. They do this by protecting us from damage caused by free radicals, which can injure healthy cells and tissues. The body produces free radicals in the normal course of energy production, but there are also substances in our surrounding environment—certain chemicals, smoke, pollutants, solar radiation—that trigger the production of free radicals. Don't underestimate the threat free radicals pose to our health and well-being. Scientists now believe that free radicals are causal factors in nearly every known disease, from heart disease to arthritis to cancer to cataracts. In fact, free radicals are a major culprit in the aging process itself.

By controlling free radicals, antioxidants can make the difference between life and death, as well as influence how fast and how well we age. The more you understand about antioxidants and how they work, the more you will understand and appreciate the profound role they play in keeping you healthy and happy. Their role in the human body is nothing less than miraculous.

There is overwhelming scientific evidence demonstrating that those of us who eat a diet rich in antioxidants and take antioxidant supplements will live longer, healthier lives. In this book I will tell you about some of these exciting, groundbreaking studies, and I will show you how to use these discoveries to improve your life *right now*. Starting today, you can halt and even reverse many of the age-related problems that can arise—and make life so miserable—when our bodies suffer from an overabundance of free radicals and a deficit of antioxidants.

Scientists have known about the existence of antioxidants for decades, but until very recently, we have not fully understood what they do, how they do it, and how to tap their incredible power. Thanks to work performed at the Packer Lab at the University of California at Berkeley, and in other labs around the world, we have found the answers to these questions, and we now know how to maximize and harness the lifesaving, life-extending power of antioxidants.

Introducing the antioxidant network

Until recently, scientists believed that each antioxidant worked separately in the body, independently of the others. We now know this isn't true—there is a dynamic interplay among certain key antioxidants. I refer to this interplay as the *antioxidant network* and I refer to the chemical players as the *network antioxidants*. These special network antioxidants work together in our bodies to strengthen us and protect us from disease.

Although there are literally hundreds of antioxidants, only five appear to be network antioxidants: *Vitamins C* and *E, glutathione, lipoic acid,* and *Coenzyme Q10 (Co Q10)*. Vitamins C and E are not produced in the body but must be obtained through food. Glutathione, lipoic acid, and Co Q10 are produced by the body, but levels of these antioxidants decline as we age. That is why we need to supplement all of them.

In the Packer Lab, we have discovered that network antioxidants have special powers that set them apart from other antioxidants. What makes network antioxidants so special is that they can greatly enhance the power of one another. As a result, they are particularly effective in slowing down the aging process and boosting the body's ability to fight disease. The antioxidant network is a shield that protects the body against the forces that age us before our time and rob years from our lives.

Not so long ago, the diseases of aging were accepted as unfortunate but inevitable facts of life. At the turn of the last century, the average life span was a meager forty-seven years. Today no one blinks when we live into our eighties or nineties, and some scientists think that within a few generations, many of us will live well into our hundreds. You probably aren't surprised because you've seen what modern medicine, better sanitation, and improved nutrition can do to extend life span; however, you've probably also noticed that although people are living longer, too many are plagued by chronic diseases that not only hamper their ability to make the most of these added years, but sometimes even seem to make them a curse. A longer life doesn't have to be this way.

Thanks to our new understanding of antioxidants and the role of the antioxidant network, we can live not just longer, but live well, in bodies that stay healthy, strong, and vigorous, with minds that are alert and memories that are intact. I am not talking about just adding years to our lives; I am talking about adding life to our years.

We now know that the key to preventing disease and extending life is as simple as maintaining the right level and combination of antioxidants in our bodies. I call this the *antioxidant advantage,* and I will show you how it can help you to achieve long life and optimal health.

For more than three decades, the Packer Lab has been a mecca for the best and brightest researchers in the field of antioxidants from around the world. When people ask me to describe the Packer Lab, I tell them it's a lot like working in the United Nations. There are days when I walk into my laboratory and am greeted with "Good morning" in sixteen different languages. I am very proud that my laboratory has trained many of the world's finest scientists, and that today there are Packer Lab alumni in top research centers from London to Tel Aviv to Tokyo and to nearly every place in between.

I am particularly proud of my laboratory's leadership role in discovering how antioxidants work together in the body, but we are probably best known for our discovery of the special role played by a newly identified antioxidant, lipoic acid, the most versatile and powerful antioxidant in the network. Lipoic acid greatly enhances the power of all the other antioxidants in the body. For more than two decades, lipoic acid has been used safely and successfully in Europe as a treatment for complications of diabetes. Research in my laboratory has shown that lipoic acid may offer powerful protection against both stroke and heart disease. As I will be explaining later in the book, since you can't get enough lipoic acid through food alone, if you're not taking lipoic acid supplements, you're not tapping the full power of the antioxidant network.

The first time many of you may have heard about lipoic acid was when I was interviewed about my work on ABC's *World News Tonight* last year. The two-minute segment on lipoic acid generated so many calls, letters, and visits to the Packer Lab web site for more information that I recognized the need to share this lifesaving information with the public.

I have also been a pioneer in the study of vitamin E, an antioxidant that is breaking new ground nearly every day. You've probably noticed it's hard to pick up the newspaper without reading about a new way that vitamin E promotes health. Vitamin E can protect us from such diseases as Alzheimer's disease, heart disease, and several common types of cancer. And if you have also grown accustomed to seeing advertisements in sports and fitness magazines touting the importance of antioxidants for athletes, it is because twenty years ago my lab discovered that exercise depletes the body of vitamin E and other antioxidants and that they have to be replaced if exercise is to produce the desired effects. Experiments in my lab have also produced some tantalizing results that suggest vitamin E can even extend our life span.

We have also discovered that some nonnetwork antioxidants and even some substances that are not antioxidants can enhance the effectiveness of one or more network antioxidants. These include members of the flavonoid family, a group of several thousand phytochemicals (plant-based chemicals). There are fifty different common flavonoid compounds found in fruits, vegetables, and beverages, including green tea and red wine. Selenium, a mineral that strengthens the network antioxidants, is an example of a nonantioxidant that is a true miracle maker.

There are scores of other bona fide antioxidants that do not interact with the network, but nevertheless help its mission by reducing the free radical load in the body. These helper antioxidants include members of the carotenoid family, a group of coloring agents found in foods, especially in dark-green leafy vegetables and orange and yellow fruits and vegetables.

In *The Antioxidant Miracle,* I will not only be reporting on work performed in my own lab, I will also be telling you about the work of my distinguished colleagues. Until now, these discoveries have been described mainly in scholarly books and journals written for other scientists. In *The Antioxidant Miracle,* I will be passing this groundbreaking information on to you. Scientists all over the world are investigating the role of antioxidants in extending life and preventing disease. For example:

* Are you getting sick more often than you used to? As we age, immune function declines, making us vulnerable to disease. Tufts University researchers have found that antioxidants can rejuvenate an aging immune system.

* Do you think that you have bad genes? Many of us inherit the tendency to develop cancer and other diseases. The good news is that antioxidants can "turn off" these bad genes and greatly reduce our risk of developing hereditary diseases.

* Do you feel that you're not as sharp as you used to be? Numerous studies suggest that antioxidants can prevent and perhaps even reverse age-related memory loss and mental problems.

* Do you have a child with attention deficit disorder (ADD), or do you have ADD yourself? There is growing evidence that antioxidants can improve concentration and focus in people suffering from ADD.

* Do you wake up with aches and pains? Antioxidants can relieve the symptoms of arthritis and other inflammatory conditions.

* Are you at risk for developing heart disease? Antioxidants such as vitamin E and Co Q10 are being used successfully to treat heart disease.

* Do you have brown spots and other signs of sun-damaged skin? Antioxidants can prevent and even erase these telltale signs of age while also protecting against skin cancer.

The Antioxidant Miracle will explain the science behind the miracle and show you how to make the miracle work for you.

In Parts One to Three of this book, I will review the latest scientific information on antioxidants in simple, easy-to-understand language. In Part Four, The Packer Plan—Making the Antioxidant Miracle Work for You, I will describe the Packer Plan, a comprehensive three-part program featuring:

* **An antioxidant feast**   Common, everyday foods found at your local supermarket and greengrocer contain hundreds of lifesaving antioxidants. The Packer Plan will show you how easy it is to maintain your antioxidant advantage by eating the right foods.

* **Your supplement regimen**   The Packer Plan offers a state-of-the-art supplement regimen that is designed to keep your body strong, your brain sharp, and your antioxidant network working at its peak. In addition to a basic supplement program that is suitable for most people, I will also be tailoring my supplement regimen to accommodate people with special needs, such as smokers, diabetics, people with a family history of cancer or heart disease, menopausal women, athletes, and even picky eaters.

* **Antioxidants for healthy, beautiful skin**   The Packer Lab is the world's leading research center on antioxidants and skin. From

our research, we have learned that it is as important to replenish antioxidants on the outside as it is on the inside. The Packer Plan includes an antioxidant skin-care regimen that not only prevents skin cancer but can slow down and even reverse wrinkles, fine lines, and other signs of aging.

Can you get enough antioxidant protection from food alone?

Since all the network antioxidants can be found in food, you may wonder why I recommend that you also take supplements. Eating an antioxidant-rich diet is an important part of the Packer Plan, but it is virtually impossible to get the optimal amount of antioxidants through food alone. For example, the Packer Plan recommends taking 500 I.U. of vitamin E daily. In order to get 500 I.U. of vitamin E from food alone, you would have to eat more than 100 pounds of broiled liver or 125 tablespoons of peanut oil—or you could take a vitamin E supplement, as I advise.

The Antioxidant Miracle can change and extend your life. More than 70 percent of Americans will die prematurely from diseases caused by or compounded by deficiencies of the antioxidant network. Thanks to the antioxidant advantage, these conditions can be prevented, controlled, and in some cases even cured. People who take even one antioxidant supplement daily can significantly reduce their risk of heart disease and prostate cancer. Can you imagine the benefits that result from supplementing the entire antioxidant network? In *The Antioxidant Miracle,* I will be showing you how to do that, and explaining why the benefits will astonish you.

As we move into the new millennium, the Antioxidant Miracle makes it possible for each of us to have greater control over our health, and ultimately our destiny, than we ever had before. We now have the power to prevent and perhaps even eradicate many of the degenerative diseases that were once considered an inevitable part of aging.

This is a true miracle.

2

The Antioxidant
Network in Action
Vitamins C and E, Co Q10,
Lipoic Acid, Glutathione

The Antioxidant Miracle has been a long time in the making. The discovery of the antioxidant network—the five special antioxidants that work together in spectacular synergy—is the culmination of nearly one-half century of research spanning the lives and careers of many distinguished scientists. Thanks to the work of these creative pioneers, we now know that antioxidants can protect us from heart disease, cancer, and diabetes and enable us to live longer lives in healthier bodies. I was able to build on the work of these pioneers as well as my own decades of research to develop the network antioxidant concept, a breakthrough in our understanding of how antioxidants work. Our new understanding of the antioxidant network now enables us to harness the full potential of the Antioxidant Miracle.

I have been fortunate to be a part of the Antioxidant Miracle from the very beginning, when a small group of scientists created a new field of study: cell biology. Unlike traditional biologists, who study whole organisms and their relationship to nature, we cell biologists focus on the cell, which is the basic (if not quite the smallest) unit of all living

14

organisms. The antioxidant story could not be told until the science of cell biology matured because the Antioxidant Miracle occurs on the cellular level, and until the past few decades, it could not be observed, let alone understood or explained.

You and I and every animal and human being are made up of trillions of cells. Similar cells combine to form tissues, and similar tissues combine to form organs. When I was a biology major at Brooklyn College in the late 1940s, we were scarcely aware of the existence of antioxidants, let alone the critical role they played at the cellular level. Scientists did know from long experience that if we didn't get enough vitamin C in our diet, we could develop scurvy. Scientists also knew about the existence of another vitamin, vitamin E, but no one knew what it did.

Other scientists—food chemists—were also looking at these vitamins because they thought vitamins might be good food preservatives. They appeared to prevent the process of oxidation, which causes fat to become rancid.

To understand the process of oxidation, all you have to do is think about what goes on in your kitchen every day. At the end of a meal, you wrap up leftovers to keep them from spoiling. One reason wrapping food works is that, at least for a while, it keeps oxygen from attacking that uneaten drumstick or grapefruit half. Food chemists had figured out that these vitamins protected food from this oxidation process, and so they began to refer to them as *antioxidants*. Of course, we cell biologists weren't particularly interested in what the food chemists were doing because we didn't think their work was relevant to ours. It didn't occur to anyone that the same process was occurring within our own bodies. As a result, it took a long time for us to put together what must now strike you as being as simple as two plus two.

The secret world of the cell

In the early and mid-1950s, we were eager to begin our exploration of the uncharted world of the cell, but we were hampered by archaic technology and tight money. At many universities, science was still at the bottom of the funding totem pole, and finding money for our experiments was almost as challenging as testing our hypotheses. But all that was about to change. In 1957, the Soviet Union launched *Sputnik*, the world's first orbiting satellite, and suddenly Americans were fearful of lagging behind Russia in science. Practically overnight, the government began to invest more money in basic scientific research and education, and many spectacular technological advancements resulted.

From my perspective, one of the most important was the development of the electron microscope. Many thousands of times more powerful than the old-fashioned light microscope, the electron microscope propelled cell biology into the twentieth century. Without it, there would be no Antioxidant Miracle.

I do not want to give you the impression that the history of cell biology begins with the electron microscope. Indeed, the light microscope did help us learn a lot. The light microscope enabled us to see the basic, larger structures within the cell and gave us a surprisingly sophisticated knowledge of what a cell looked like. For example, we were able to see that every cell had a protective covering on the outside and a structure on the inside. We called the covering the *cell membrane,* and we called the internal structure the *nucleus.* We could even make out some of the other main cell structures, but we could only speculate about what they did and how they did it. The electron microscope brought everything into sharp focus. For the first time, we could see the smallest components of the cell and study how they interacted and worked.

Before the electron microscope, we knew about the existence of tiny structures within the cell called *mitochondria,* which converted nutrients into cellular energy in a process called *biological oxidation.* Now, with the electron microscope, we could see in breathtaking detail these miniature cellular powerhouses in action. It was the study of biological oxidation that finally revealed the importance of antioxidants.

Free radicals

As I quickly learned, oxygen can be a dangerous friend. The human body requires ample amounts of oxygen for metabolism, the breakdown of nutrients to create the energy for growth and other body activities. Energy is essential for every physical activity, from breathing to thinking, from having sex to keeping our hearts beating. Oxygen is the fuel that turns on energy production. Without oxygen, we could not make energy. Yet the production of energy can wreak havoc in the body because it also produces free radicals. Free radicals are unstable molecules that can damage cell structures and can ultimately lead to cancer, heart disease, and numerous other illnesses. As I will explain later, Alzheimer's disease, Parkinson's disease, diabetes, cataracts, arthritis, and many other ailments associated with aging are caused or aggravated by free radicals.

The key to good health is to maintain the right balance between antioxidants and free radicals. That is the job of the body's antioxidant defense network.

How antioxidants work with free radicals

The job of defending the body against free radicals falls to the antioxidant defense system, a group of compounds that are uniquely qualified to disarm free radicals before they can attack their target tissue. Antioxidants are the free radical police of the body, on call whenever necessary to "quench" free radicals wherever they may be, so that they cannot spread their destruction to other cells.

There are literally hundreds of naturally occurring antioxidants. Some antioxidants are produced by the body, while others must be obtained from food or supplements.

When an antioxidant encounters a free radical, it engulfs it, and the free radical then joins its molecular structure. The antioxidant itself becomes a free radical. So what have you gained? These newly created free radicals are relatively weak and are not likely to do further harm. Therefore, you are sparing your cells and tissues from the destructive path of a free radical out of control.

Within the body, there is a dynamic interplay between five key antioxidants: vitamins C and E, Co Q10, lipoic acid, and glutathione. These are the network antioxidants. These special antioxidants work together to bolster and strengthen the entire system. When combined, they greatly enhance the activity of one another, helping the body to maintain the right antioxidant balance. In the Packer Lab, we have discovered that network antioxidants have special powers not shared by the others. What makes network antioxidants special is that they can "recycle," or regenerate, one another after they have quenched a free radical, vastly extending their antioxidant power.

Here's an example of how network antioxidants work together. When vitamin E disarms a free radical, it becomes a weak free radical itself. But unlike bad free radicals, the vitamin E radical can be recycled, or turned back into an antioxidant, by vitamin C or Coenzyme Q10. These network antioxidants will donate electrons to vitamin E, bringing it back to its antioxidant state. The same scenario occurs when vitamin C or glutathione defuses a free radical and becomes a weak free radical in the process. These antioxidants can be recycled back to their antioxidant form by lipoic acid or vitamin C.

The primary job of the antioxidant network is to prevent antioxidants from being lost through oxidation. As one network antioxidant saves the other, the cycle continues, ensuring that the body will maintain the right antioxidant balance.

This particular scenario—antioxidant meets free radical, antioxidant overtakes the free radical, antioxidant becomes a "friendly" free radical, antioxidant is recycled by another network antioxidant—occurs countless times in the body in the blink of an eye. It's virtually impossible for us to comprehend how often or how fast this all happens, but to give you a rough idea of the frequency with which antioxidants are called into action by the body, consider this: my colleague, Bruce Ames, a well-known scientist in the field of antioxidants, estimates that the number of oxidative hits daily to DNA per human cell is about 10,000. Now multiply that by the trillions of cells in the body, and you can begin to understand the magnitude of these numbers. If you do not replenish the lost antioxidants through food and supplements, you will be leaving yourself vulnerable to further damage.

Although the network antioxidants work in synergy, each has a unique niche in the cell where it exerts protective action. For example, the cell membrane is made primarily of fats or lipids, but the cell itself is filled with water. Fat-soluble vitamin E and Co Q10 protect the fatty portion of the cell membrane from free radical attack. But don't count on them to protect the watery portions of the cell, or blood, which is primarily water. These areas are accessible only to the water-soluble antioxidants such as vitamin C and glutathione.

There is only one antioxidant we know of that is allowed in both watery and fatty areas—lipoic acid. Lipoic acid is unique in that it can function in both zones and can regenerate both water-soluble (vitamin C and glutathione) and fat-soluble (vitamin E) antioxidants.

The important thing to remember is that each of the network antioxidants is greater than the sum of its parts, and that when combined, they create a juggernaut against the lethal forces of oxidation.

Below, I give a brief review of each network antioxidant, and I describe how it works separately and together with the others.

The network antioxidants

Lipoic Acid

Until recently, lipoic acid was considered a relatively unimportant antioxidant, not worthy of a second glance. If people are taking a closer look at lipoic acid these days, I am proud to say it is as a result of work performed at the Packer Lab showing that lipoic acid is the most versatile and powerful antioxidant in the entire antioxidant defense network.

Relatively new to the United States, lipoic acid has been used in Europe safely and effectively for more than three decades in the treatment of complications from diabetes. My research has revealed that lipoic acid may also offer significant protection against stroke, the third leading cause of death in the Western world, and heart disease. Lipoic acid is unique in that it is the only antioxidant that can significantly boost the levels of glutathione, another key network antioxidant that is instrumental in ridding the body of toxins. Since lipoic acid can recycle glutathione, it is important because, when taken orally, glutathione is not well absorbed by the body and most of it goes to waste. My laboratory has shown that lipoic acid can boost glutathione levels in cells by an impressive 30 percent. When you take lipoic acid, you are not only getting all the benefits of lipoic acid, but you are in effect getting an additional dose of glutathione.

Vitamin E

Vitamin E, the body's primary fat-soluble antioxidant, must be obtained from food or supplements. Compared to glutathione or vitamin C, there is only a tiny amount of vitamin E in the cells, yet it is one of the most important and well studied of all the antioxidants. Vitamin E travels through the body in molecules called *lipoproteins* and protects them from oxidation. The oxidation of lipoproteins is believed to be the first step in the formation of atherosclerosis, hardening of the arteries, which can lead to heart disease. Recent studies have shown that vitamin E can prevent heart disease, reduce the risk of prostate cancer, and even slow down the progression of Alzheimer's disease.

Vitamin C

Championed by Nobel Laureate Linus Pauling, who claimed vitamin C was the cure for the common cold, vitamin C is a water-soluble antioxidant. (Dr. Pauling may have been right, but for the wrong reasons, which I'll discuss later.) Vitamin C is not produced by the body and must be obtained through food or supplements. Vitamin C is a potent free radical quencher, and it is essential for a strong immune system. Studies performed by my colleagues at the University of California have shown that people who take vitamin C supplements live longer, healthier lives than those who don't.

Coenzyme Q10

Coenzyme Q10 (Co Q10) is a fat-soluble molecule that works synergistically with vitamin E in the antioxidant cycle to protect the fatty part of the cell from free radical attack. Numerous studies document that Co Q10 is an effective treatment for heart failure, angina, and high blood pressure. It is also being investigated as a treatment for cancer and age-related brain diseases such as Parkinson's and Alzheimer's.

Glutathione

The most abundant antioxidant in the network is glutathione, which is produced by the body from three amino acids found in food: *glutamic acid, cysteine,* and *glycine.* Glutathione is found in virtually every cell and is an important weapon in the battle against free radicals. When we reach the age of forty, our production of glutathione begins to decline; it can drop almost 20 percent by the time we are sixty. At any age, low levels of glutathione have been linked to premature death and disease. It is essential to keep your levels of glutathione high.

Monitoring the health of your cells

In addition to controlling free radicals, antioxidants play an even more critical role in the maintenance of health: They help control our genes. Let me explain why this quality is so important and what it has to do with the Antioxidant Miracle.

Most of you have a basic understanding of how physical characteristics, such as eye or hair color, are passed on to your children through your genes. What you may not fully appreciate is that your genes do more than carry your physical blueprint. They also contain the mechanism for keeping your body healthy and strong.

Your cells cannot think for themselves; they rely on genes to tell them what to do. The DNA that is contained within each of our genes carries a vast library of instructions that regulate all cellular activity. For example, when your immune system is confronted with a dangerous virus that could spread disease if it were allowed to live, it is your genes that alert the immune system to produce special cells to kill the virus. When healthy cells are damaged by a virus or turn cancerous, it is your genes that instruct the bad cells to self-destruct before they can spread to other healthy cells. Think of your genes as the ultimate pharmacy, the keeper of a secret formula that is designed to keep you healthy and functioning at peak capacity. When you are in trouble, it is up to your genes to rescue you by telling your cells what to do.

Clearly, genes play a critical role in controlling our ability to fight disease. One of the questions that I have spent my life studying is, What, if anything, controls our genes?

This vital job falls to the antioxidant network.

I mentioned earlier that antioxidants protect the DNA in genes from free radical attack, but we discovered that is not the only job they perform. We have learned that antioxidants also regulate the expression of genes. In fact, I believe that the single most important scientific breakthrough of the Packer Lab is our discovery that antioxidants switch genes on and off in accordance with what the body requires.

The antioxidant network functions as our personal physician, constantly monitoring the health of our cells. If the network detects a problem in a particular area, it will turn on the appropriate genes to produce the appropriate response. The network sends signals to our genes, which in turn tell our cells whether to eat, live, die, or reproduce. By controlling the trillions of cells that comprise our bodies, the antioxidant network controls every aspect of our lives.

When we are young, our bodies hear the messages of the antioxidant network loud and clear. As a result, we function at an optimal level. But as we age, the antioxidant network becomes overwhelmed with work. One reason is that our antioxidant levels decline. In addition, pollution, smoking, poor diet, and other unhealthy influences may have added to the free radical challenge confronting the network. The result is that the network becomes less able to function as the body's personal physician. The messages it receives and sends become confused. It misses problems and fails to respond when it should. Under these conditions, diseases can take hold.

Keeping your antioxidant network strong is the only way to give your personal physician the tools it needs to maintain youthful health and vitality. Replenishing the body's network antioxidants with daily supplements as I recommend in the Packer Plan offers new hope in preventing the epidemics of cancer, heart disease, and other illnesses that typically strike later in life when antioxidant defenses are down. By following the Packer Plan, you can reasonably expect to lead a longer, healthier life.

Knowledge is power, and for the first time in human history, we have both the knowledge and the power to make a significant inroad in eradicating disease, maintaining health, and ultimately controlling our destiny. That is what *The Antioxidant Miracle* is all about.

3

Free Radicals
Both Enemy and Friend

Before you can fully understand *The Antioxidant Miracle,* you need to know more about the nemesis of antioxidants: free radicals. As the adage goes, wherever there is smoke, there is fire. Similarly, wherever there is disease and destruction, there are free radicals. The flip side is that wherever there is life, there are free radicals. We could not exist without them. We have only just begun to fully appreciate the role of free radicals in the body.

Every time we try to remember a fact or are sexually aroused or are battling a cold, we are putting free radicals to good use. Free radicals perform many critical functions in our bodies, from controlling the flow of blood through our arteries, to fighting infection, to keeping our brains sharp and in focus.

Similar to antioxidants, some free radicals at low levels are signaling molecules—that is, they are responsible for turning on and off genes. Some free radicals, such as nitric oxide and superoxide, are produced in very high amounts by our immune cells to "poison" viruses and bacteria. Some free radicals kill cancer cells, and in fact, many cancer drugs are actually designed to increase the production of free radicals in the body. The role of nitric oxide is so important that in 1998, the Nobel Prize in Physiology and Medicine was awarded to the scientists who discovered nitric oxide's role as a signaling molecule in the cardiovascular system.

Clearly, we need free radicals for our survival. Yet, in less than a split second, free radicals can turn on us, make us sick, and age us before our time. Whether it is a sunburn, a heart attack, a stroke, or an inflammatory illness such as arthritis, free radicals are a factor in either the onset or progression of these conditions. Even the aging process itself is linked to free radicals.

Free radicals are everywhere

In order to understand what free radicals are, you need to know a bit about the human cell, where the tug-of-war between free radicals and antioxidants is played out every second of every day. Like everything else in the universe, cells are composed of smaller units called *atoms*. Each atom contains a center or nucleus that is surrounded by electrons. Two or more atoms may bind together by sharing electrons. Biological oxidation, the process of making energy, involves moving electrons from one oxygen molecule to the next. However, sometimes an electron escapes. This "free" electron is called a free radical.

Free radicals constantly form almost everywhere in the body at an astonishing rate. If free radicals are not quickly trapped, they can cause a great deal of trouble. Free radicals can attack and oxidize DNA, the genetic material that controls cell growth and development, which can increase the likelihood of cancer. When these unstable molecules target fat molecules traveling in the bloodstream, they set the stage for heart disease and stroke. Therefore, free radicals can promote the downward spiral of disease and premature aging.

Free radicals fast-forward the aging process

Many of you are taking antioxidants because you want to look and feel younger. This is not just wishful thinking. Maintaining the antioxidant advantage—that is, keeping free radicals in check—may be one of the most effective ways to slow down the aging process.

What has become known as the *free radical theory of aging* was first proposed by Dr. Denham Harman in 1954, a postdoctoral researcher at Berkeley who was studying the effects of radiation on human biological systems. The United States was in the middle of the Cold War with the Soviet Union, and there was very real fear that it would heat up into a nuclear war. Researchers such as Dr. Harman were commissioned by the government to invent an effective antidote to radiation poisoning that would result from an atomic attack. What makes radiation exposure so dangerous is that it triggers the production of the lethal *hydroxyl radical,* the most powerful and deadly free radical known. This free radical is usually made when water comes in contact with ionizing radiation. The hydroxyl radical is highly reactive, destroying everything in its path. Once it is created, it is nearly impossible to stop.

Dr. Harman was the first to make the connection between free radicals produced by radiation exposure and the free radicals produced through normal energy production in the body. He noticed that mild radiation poisoning produced symptoms that were similar to premature aging and hypothesized that in aging, free radicals are responsible for producing the same effects, only over a longer time.

When I first heard Dr. Harman explain his free radical theory of aging more than thirty years ago, his ideas coincided with my own beliefs. I had already reached the conclusion that our standard method of researching the aging process—studying young versus old animals—was sadly outmoded. I believed that the key to unraveling the mysteries of aging lay in our cells—specifically, through enhancing our understanding of biological oxidation, how cells use oxygen to produce energy. This fundamental activity is carried out by every cell in the body, and it seemed to me that it would somehow be relevant to explain why and how we age. When Dr. Harman proposed that a by-product of biological oxidation—free radicals—was instrumental in aging, it made great sense to me, and it still does.

Through the years, Dr. Harman has become a good friend and a valued colleague. Now in his eighties, this modest, soft-spoken scientist is still trim and active, and he is a frequent speaker at gerontological meetings. Dr. Harman is vigilant about taking his antioxidants, and he watches what he eats and exercises regularly.

While we can't stop the years from passing—or our bodies from growing older—we can use antioxidants to help minimize the damage inflicted by free radicals, thereby slowing down the process.

Free radicals not only age the body from the inside, but from the outside as well. When ultraviolet radiation from the sun hits the skin, it excites a molecule on the skin's surface that reacts with oxygen to form singlet oxygen. Singlet oxygen is potentially dangerous because it can promote the formation of free radicals.

Ozone, an oxygen molecule with an extra electron, is another skin ager. Ozone is present in cigarette smoke and automobile exhaust. Although it is not a free radical, it promotes the formation of free radicals. Ozone not only attacks the skin, but when it is breathed into the lungs, it can destroy the fluid lining of the lungs, the nasal passages, and the buccal oral cavity.

Free radicals and stroke

Stroke is an example of how free radicals do their dirty work, and how they can make a bad situation even worse. A stroke occurs when blood flow is cut off or restricted to a particular region of the brain. It could be caused by a blood clot, or by a piece of debris that breaks off from an atherosclerotic plaque and blocks the artery delivering blood and oxygen to the brain. Whatever the cause, the results can be devastating. You may be surprised to know that much of the actual damage to the brain does not occur when it is being deprived of blood and oxygen, but immediately following the stroke, when the blood flow is restored. This is called *reperfusion injury*. When it happens, there is a burst in production of superoxide free radicals that can attack nearby tissue, resulting in permanent brain damage.

The situation can get even more serious if in the process of damaging brain tissue, iron is released into sites where it is normally tightly bound or controlled. Iron is the most abundant mineral in the body and it is vital for life, but iron is not allowed to roam freely throughout the body. It is held tightly bound to proteins, carried to tissues where it is deposited into storage sites, and closely guarded.

The body goes to great pains to contain iron. Free iron—that is, iron that is not bound to a protein—is potentially very dangerous because it can trigger free radical reactions. More free radicals are the last thing brain tissue needs to contend with after a stroke. High accumulations of iron in the brain have also been associated with degenerative diseases such as Alzheimer's and Parkinson's. Not surprisingly, there have also been several studies that have linked high blood levels of free iron to an increased risk of heart disease and stroke.

Free radicals and heart disease

Free radicals are involved in both the onset and the progression of heart disease in several different ways. When you think of heart disease, you undoubtedly think of chest pain or a heart attack, but heart disease begins long before the first symptoms are ever felt. Heart disease begins years earlier with the oxidation of LDL (low-density lipoproteins), also known as "bad" cholesterol. This is the first domino to fall in a long sequence of events that lead to the formation of plaque in the arteries delivering blood to the heart. The process can take many years, but if the artery becomes clogged with plaque, the result can be a sudden loss of blood and oxygen to the heart, or a heart attack. As with a stroke, much of the damage that occurs to the heart muscle from a heart attack is caused by a burst of free radicals after the blood flow is resumed.

Recently we have learned of another way in which free radicals can promote atherosclerosis (hardening of the arteries), and how one free radical in particular, *nitric oxide,* may play a central role. Although it is essential for normal blood circulation, excess nitric oxide can be very dangerous and is believed to be a factor in heart disease and stroke. In order to have good circulatory health, the body must maintain the right balance of nitric oxide, and doing that job falls to the network antioxidants and their boosters.

Free radicals and chronic inflammation

Inflammation is caused by the overproduction of free radicals in a specific area of the body. It is responsible for about 30 percent of all cancers and is a contributing factor, if not the cause, of numerous other medical problems.

Most of you know that exposure to asbestos can lead to a type of lung cancer called mesothelioma. What is not widely known, however, is that asbestos leads to chronic inflammation of the lung tissue, which in turn promotes the proliferation of free radicals. This leads to lung fibrosis, which can affect proper breathing. Here's what happens. The asbestos molecule is an unwieldy structure with jagged edges. When it is inhaled into the airways, the cells of the immune system recognize there is a problem, and they send out a legion of special cells called *leukocytes* to deal with it. Think of leukocytes as microscopic fire engines dispatched to the scene of a fire, but the only problem is, in the case of asbestos, the fire never stops burning. The asbestos molecule is simply too big and awkwardly shaped for the leukocytes to control, but they never stop trying. One of the weapons that immune cells use to attack a foreign invader is free radicals. So the leukocytes become locked in a losing battle with the asbestos molecules to gain back control of the affected lung tissue. All the while, they are spewing forth free radicals, which paradoxically are causing further damage. This creates a wound that never heals and that is chronically inflamed. After years of bombardment, the result can be lung cancer.

The inflammatory response is also a factor in arthritis, an umbrella term for more than 100 different diseases that produce either inflammation of connective tissue (the joints and tendons) or degeneration of the articular cartilage, a wearing down of the protective covering that cushions the ends of bones, allowing bones to rub together without causing damage to the joints.

When joints become arthritic, they become inflamed and enlarged, interfering with the normal flow of blood. For example, in the case of an arthritic knee, when you bend the knee, you cut off blood flow to the area. As you may remember from my description of stroke, when blood flow is cut off, it sets in motion a chain of events that will lead to a burst of free radicals when the blood flow returns, which is precisely what happens when you release the knee. The proliferation of free radicals causes the area to become even more inflamed, contributing to the degeneration of the joint, which becomes more swollen and worn down.

Free radicals can be enemies or friends, but we have to interact with them the right way, or they can quickly turn against us. The key is to maintain the antioxidant advantage, the optimal balance between free radicals and antioxidants. We can achieve the antioxidant advantage by consuming adequate amounts of antioxidants in the form of food and supplements, and by limiting exposure to "pro-oxidants" in the environment that can harm us.

PART TWO

The Miracle Within

Nature's Super Antioxidant Defense Network

4

Lipoic Acid

The Universal Antioxidant

※ L ipoic acid offers powerful protection against three common ailments of aging: stroke, heart disease, and cataracts.

※ Lipoic acid strengthens memory and prevents brain aging.

※ Lipoic acid boosts the entire antioxidant defense network. By taking lipoic acid, you are in effect increasing your levels of vitamins E and C, glutathione, and Coenzyme Q10.

※ Lipoic acid is new to the United States. It has been used safely and effectively in Europe for more than two decades to prevent and relieve the complications of diabetes.

※ Lipoic acid turns off bad genes that can accelerate aging and cause cancer.

※ Lipoic acid is reported to reverse mushroom poisoning of the liver, which is usually lethal. It has been used successfully to treat other liver diseases such as hepatitis C.

※ *RDA:* None.

* *The Packer Plan:* 100 milligrams daily (50 milligrams in the A.M. and 50 milligrams in the P.M.).
* *Sources:* Synthesized by the body. Present in small amounts in potatoes, spinach, and red meat.

For nearly a decade, much of my research has focused on lipoic acid, a truly remarkable antioxidant that has forever changed the way scientists think of antioxidants. It was from my work with lipoic acid that I was able to develop the concept of an antioxidant network more fully, and to gain greater understanding of the extraordinary role that antioxidants play far beyond that of the body's free radical police.

Lipoic acid is a *superantioxidant* that breaks many of the rules regarding antioxidant behavior. In fact, if I were to invent an ideal antioxidant, it would closely resemble lipoic acid, which does everything an antioxidant should do and more. Here are some of the ways lipoic acid is special. Lipoic acid:

IS INCREDIBLY VERSATILE   Each cell has a fatty barrier in its membrane that prevents the water-soluble components outside from mixing with the water-soluble components inside. Other network antioxidants are either fat- or water-soluble, which means they are not allowed access to all parts of the cell. Because of its unique structure, lipoic acid is allowed into both the fatty and watery portions of the cell, which greatly enhances its ability to trap free radicals wherever they may be.

CAN RECYCLE ALL OF THE NETWORK ANTIOXIDANTS   As you may recall, when an antioxidant "quenches" a free radical, it turns into a free radical itself. When this happens, it is lost to the antioxidant network, unless it is restored to its antioxidant form. Lipoic acid is the only antioxidant that can recycle all of the network antioxidants: vitamin E, Coenzyme Q10, glutathione, and vitamin C. Lipoic acid is the antioxidant's antioxidant.

IS CRITICAL FOR ENERGY PRODUCTION   Lipoic acid helps break down sugar for the production of ATP, the fuel produced by cells to run the body. In fact, without lipoic acid, cells cannot utilize energy and they will shut down.

REGENERATES ITSELF   Lipoic acid taps into the same machinery involved in cellular energy production to recycle itself from its free radical form back to its antioxidant form, the only antioxidant that can perform this feat. This ability to restore itself (and other antioxidants) is one of the reasons that lipoic acid is so important in maintaining our antioxidant advantage.

Is lipoic acid a vitamin?

Until recently, lipoic acid was nature's best-kept secret. Lipoic acid was first discovered in 1937 by scientists who observed that bacteria required a component of potato extract to grow in culture. This unknown nutrient was called "potato growth factor," but no one knew what it was, what it did, or whether it was even important for humans.

In 1951, biochemist Lester Reed isolated lipoic acid and mapped out its molecular structure. This was no easy task. It took 10 tons of beef liver to produce a scant 30 milligrams of lipoic acid! By now, researchers knew that lipoic acid was an essential nutrient for growth, and some thought that it might even be a vitamin. A vitamin is a nutrient that is necessary for the normal functioning of the body but is not produced by the body and must be obtained from food. It was later discovered that lipoic acid is produced by animals, humans, and even plants, but in minuscule quantities, disqualifying it from gaining vitamin status.

However, the more I learn about lipoic acid, the more I believe that it should be given vitamin status. The primary reason is that lipoic acid production declines with age. By midlife, we may be producing enough lipoic acid to meet our body's most basic needs, but not enough to get the full range of benefits that lipoic acid has to offer. Therefore, it is essential to supplement lipoic acid from other sources. Although I strongly believe in the importance of a good diet, as I discuss in chapter 13, it is extremely difficult to get enough lipoic acid from food since it is present in such tiny amounts: It takes 7 pounds of spinach to produce just 1 milligram of lipoic acid. Clearly, it is impossible to ingest my recommended 100 milligrams of lipoic acid daily from food alone. That is why I take a lipoic acid supplement and recommend that you do the same.

The lipoic acid story unfolded slowly over many decades. It wasn't until 1989 that lipoic acid was finally recognized as a bona fide antioxidant. Two years later, my laboratory discovered that lipoic acid was not only an integral part of the antioxidant network but was perhaps the most powerful of all the antioxidants.

We performed several remarkable experiments that brought us to this conclusion. Until recently, it had been widely believed that each antioxidant marched to the beat of a different drummer, and that there was little "cross talk" between them. In other words, each antioxidant performed its job independently of the other antioxidants.

The Packer Lab had begun to debunk this popular view. We had identified a select group of network antioxidants that worked in synergy, greatly enhancing one another's power, but we knew that we did not have the whole story. By the time I had focused my attention on lipoic acid, we had already shown that vitamin C could recycle vitamin E, and E could recycle vitamin C. We knew this because when we added either of these antioxidants to human or animal cell cultures, the level of the other antioxidant would rise—a sign that it was being recycled. The missing piece in this puzzle was which network antioxidant, if any, could recycle glutathione, the primary water-soluble antioxidant. Glutathione could be recycled through an elaborate series of chemical reactions outside of the network, but none of the known network antioxidants was able to recycle glutathione efficiently. It seemed odd that glutathione could not be easily recycled within the network, considering that it is such an important antioxidant.

Maintaining a high level of glutathione is critical for life. In fact, low glutathione levels are a marker for death at any age. Glutathione levels are drastically depleted in people with chronic illnesses such as AIDS, cancer, and autoimmune diseases (such as rheumatoid arthritis and lupus), leaving them seriously antioxidant-deficient. The problem, however, is that glutathione cannot be significantly boosted through oral supplements because most of it is broken down by digestive enzymes before it can be delivered to the cells. There are several prescription drugs that can increase glutathione levels, but none of them works particularly well. I knew instinctively that the body must have a mechanism to recycle glutathione quickly and efficiently, and I suspected that it had something to do with the newly discovered antioxidant network. I was determined to find the answer.

Although lipoic acid was not considered a major antioxidant, I had a hunch that lipoic acid might play a more important role than was then believed. Of all the antioxidants found in the body, lipoic acid was the one that was most similar in its action to glutathione. This common feature made me wonder whether lipoic acid might be able to do what the other antioxidants could not—that is, regenerate glutathione. To test my theory, my colleagues and I added lipoic acid to various types of human and animal cells in tissue culture.

We would have considered our experiments successful if we had been able to boost glutathione levels by 10 to 20 percent. Much to our excitement, in each experiment, cellular levels of glutathione rose an astonishing 30 percent. In other words, lipoic acid had succeeded where other antioxidants and drugs had failed: it could boost the levels of glutathione, a sign that it was recycling this antioxidant.

As important as test tube studies may be to biological research, the real proof is whether a theory will work *in vivo,* that is, in a living, breathing animal. In this case, my colleague Chandan Sen chose to use laboratory rats. (You may wonder why so much research is conducted on mice and rats, and what relationship these experiments have to humans. The answer is, a great deal. Rats and other rodents provide a wonderful model for the study of human beings because they develop the same diseases we do, and the pathology of these diseases is the same. These animals also rely on the same antioxidants as humans to protect them against free radicals. Therefore, these animal experiments can provide insight about the workings of our own bodies.)

In these experiments, lipoic acid was added to the chow of laboratory rats to see whether it would boost their levels of glutathione. There was a significant rise in glutathione in the lungs, liver, and blood of these animals. Lipoic acid was not only able to replenish the body's supply of precious glutathione in blood, but it did so in the tissues and cells where it was most needed.

Finally, we had found a substance that could increase glutathione, and ironically this "miracle substance" was not discovered in the laboratory of a huge drug company at a cost of billions of dollars, but it was something that nature had created and had been available to us all along. The lesson to be learned from this experience is that sometimes scientists can yield the best results when we stop trying to compete with nature or improve upon it, and instead try to understand it.

The fact that lipoic acid can boost glutathione levels so quickly and so well has important application in the prevention and treatment of numerous diseases that afflict human beings. I believe that the practice of medicine in the twenty-first century will focus less on curing disease from the outside with drugs that are foreign to our bodies, and more on empowering the body from within by boosting the disease-fighting powers of the antioxidant network.

Our discovery was also tantalizing evidence that lipoic acid was part of a much bigger story that was just beginning to unfold. We needed to further identify the role played by lipoic acid in the antioxidant network.

Lipoic acid and cataracts

Our next experiment is particularly relevant to humans because it concerns one of the most common ailments associated with aging—cataracts. A cataract is a cloudy or opaque covering that grows over the lens of the eye and is caused by free radical damage to proteins. Cataracts are so common among older people that the odds are if you live long enough, you will develop them. Cataracts are a result of years of exposure to sunlight, which can promote too many free radicals, thereby depleting the body of antioxidants.

Unlike humans who must obtain vitamin C through food or supplements, most animals can produce vitamin C on their own, with the exception of newborn animals, which cannot produce vitamin C during their first month or so of life. During these vulnerable weeks, young animals must depend on glutathione to provide their antioxidant protection. Therefore, rats that could not make glutathione would spend their first formative weeks in an antioxidant-deprived state, and as a result, would suffer specific health consequences. In many respects, these antioxidant-deficient rats share many of the same problems with older adults who are also living in an antioxidant-depressed state.

In our next experiment, we gave one group of newborn rats a drug called butathione sulphoxamine (BSO) that inhibited the production of glutathione. We gave another group of newborn rats BSO, but this time, we also gave them an injection of lipoic acid.

Newborn rats do not open their eyes until the sixth week of life, but we knew from past experiments that when these glutathione-deprived rats did open their eyes, they would all have cataracts. But the question that remained was: Would lipoic acid protect against cataracts caused by glutathione deficiency?

At the end of six weeks, as predicted, the rats that had been given the glutathione-blocking drug but had not been given lipoic acid all developed cataracts. But almost all of the rats that had been given lipoic acid supplementation had remained cataract free! Further testing revealed that glutathione levels were much higher in the eye lens of the rats treated with lipoic acid, but severely depleted in the rats not treated with lipoic acid.

It was very exciting to have finally found the antioxidant that could stimulate glutathione production. But that's not all we found. Lipoic acid had the same effect on vitamins C and E. In other words, lipoic acid supplements had not only restored glutathione, they had also boosted the levels of these other important network antioxidants. From these experiments, it became obvious that lipoic acid was an antioxidant like no other.

Lipoic acid pinch-hits for vitamin E

The experiments that truly revealed lipoic acid's pivotal role in the antioxidant network were so dramatic that there could no longer be any doubt that lipoic acid deserved a place in the antioxidant hall of fame. The results were truly spectacular.

The first experiment involved three groups of twelve-week-old mice; one group was fed a normal diet, another group was fed a vitamin E–deficient diet, and the third group was fed a vitamin E–deficient, lipoic acid–supplemented diet. After six weeks on the diet, the mice fed the normal chow developed normally, but the mice on the vitamin E–deficient diet showed signs of severe weight loss and muscle weakness. They also looked like old, scrawny, sickly mice. This was not surprising, since we already knew that severe vitamin E deficiency can cause similar symptoms in humans and animals. What was surprising was that the vitamin E–deficient mice that had been given lipoic acid showed absolutely no signs of deprivation. They were as healthy and spry as the mice fed the normal diet. Clearly, in the absence of vitamin E, lipoic acid had taken over vitamin E's functions in the body. This experiment provided positive proof of what we had already suspected. Not only was there a strong relationship between the network antioxidants, but lipoic acid played a pivotal role in this network.

Lipoic acid and stroke

Our next experiment produced even more amazing results that further reinforced my belief in the incredible power of lipoic acid, and its potential as a treatment for many different diseases, including stroke, the third leading cause of death in the United States.

Stroke is caused by a disruption in the delivery of blood and oxygen to the brain. If you're not worried about stroke, you should be. As many as 700,000 people in the United States suffer strokes each year, and 150,000 will die of them. Those who do survive a stroke often suffer physical or mental disabilities. Our studies show that lipoic acid may prove to be a weapon in the treatment of stroke, and in fact, it may help prevent strokes.

In our experiment, we induced a stroke in laboratory rats by blocking the carotid artery, which delivers blood and oxygen to the brain. After thirty minutes, blood flow was restored, and we monitored the animals for twenty-four hours. Once the oxygen was restored, there was a burst in the production of free radicals, which overwhelmed the brain's antioxidant defenses. This proved to be deadly. Within twenty-four hours after restoring oxygen, 80 percent of the rats had died.

We then repeated the experiment, with one important exception. This time, we injected the rats with lipoic acid right before we restored the normal flow of blood to the brain. Amazingly, after twenty-four hours, only 25 percent of the animals had died, and the survivors showed no sign of any problem. In fact, they had recovered completely. We know of no other antioxidant or drug that could have performed this feat.

We saw the incredible effect of lipoic acid in that it protected rats against stroke-related brain injury, but now we needed to understand the mechanism by which lipoic acid worked. In our next experiment, we looked for evidence of free radical damage in three different regions of the brain. We found that in the animals not treated with lipoic acid, there was a substantial increase in free radical–related damage in the brain, but not so in the animals treated with lipoic acid. Their brains were perfectly normal, showing no signs of the usual oxidative damage that would occur after a stroke.

Obviously, the lipoic acid injections had protected the animals against the ravages of stroke, but the question that remained was how. One of the problems in developing a treatment for stroke is that it is very difficult to design a drug that is allowed entry into the brain—that is, that can cross the so-called *brain/blood barrier.* We needed to know whether lipoic acid was one of the few substances that could actually cross the brain/blood barrier and work its magic right in the brain cells, where it was needed the most—whether it did so directly or through another member of the network.

First, we tested the brains of the treated animals for evidence of lipoic acid, and we found that lipoic acid had indeed crossed the brain/blood barrier. It had reached the brain cells in the target areas and was providing extra antioxidant support, but that's not all it did. In this time of crisis, it also boosted levels of another important network antioxidant—glutathione. In the nontreated animals, we found that the glutathione levels had plummeted after the stroke, a clear indication that the antioxidant defenses had been wiped out. In contrast, the glutathione levels in the brains of the animals treated with lipoic acid were high, a sign that they were able to successfully ward off the free radical attack. Here is yet another example of how the antioxidant network can work for our benefit, and it could literally make the difference between life and death.

Lipoic acid protects the heart

The damage that occurs to the brain after a stroke is similar to the damage that is inflicted on the heart muscle after a heart attack. Similar to a stroke, which is typically caused by a blockage in an artery delivering blood to the brain, a heart attack is usually the result of a blockage in an artery delivering blood to the heart. The result is a period of *ischemia* or oxygen deprivation followed by an explosion of free radicals when the oxygen is restored. In both cases, it is the proliferation of free radicals that exacerbates the injury.

Since lipoic acid offered significant protection against stroke, we felt that it might do the same for heart attack and devised an experiment to test our hypotheses. Our experiment utilized the so-called Langendorff beating-heart model, a procedure that allows us to study living, beating animal hearts outside of the animal's body. This not only enables us to test the effect of different drugs and therapies on beating hearts, but we can later dissect the heart and examine the full impact of our intervention on the cellular level. In our experiment, we simulated a heart attack by perfusing the beating rat hearts with a solution that did not contain oxygen. After forty minutes, we changed solutions, this time using one that contained oxygen. Based on previous experiments, we knew that if a heart is denied oxygen under these circumstances, only 20 to 25 percent of the hearts will recover and continue beating normally. The rest will suffer serious damage. When we added lipoic acid to the reperfusion solution, however, the odds were overwhelmingly tipped in favor of recovery. In fact, the recovery rate increased to almost 60 percent, more than double the rate of recovery without lipoic acid.

In a follow-up study, we fed lipoic acid to laboratory animals and then removed their hearts for further investigation. We then exposed the hearts to free radical attack. Our experiment showed that the hearts of the rats that had been fed the lipoic acid had much greater protection against free radical damage than the untreated animals. This is in keeping with our earlier experiment showing that lipoic acid can help protect heart tissue from free radical damage inflicted during a simulated heart attack.

The experiments performed in the Packer Lab clearly demonstrate how the antioxidant network in general, and lipoic acid in particular, can offer significant protection against the common ailments associated with aging, notably heart disease, stroke, and cataracts. They provide the solid scientific basis for the belief that maintaining your antioxidant advantage can help preserve health and vitality well into your later decades.

Recently, my colleague on the Berkeley campus, Prof. Bruce Ames, shared some exciting information with me. Bruce and I have had a long-standing friendship and mutual interest in the role of free radicals, oxidants, and antioxidants in the aging process. Bruce has followed the work we have been doing on lipoic acid and has conducted some interesting experiments of his own.

He and his colleagues have shown that when combined with the amino acid L-carnitine, a substance that promotes the transport of fatty acid into the cells, lipoic acid can literally rejuvenate mitochondria in old animals. As you may remember, mitochondria are the "powerhouses" of the cells, where energy is produced. As we age, our mitochondria age too, which can slow down energy production. In addition, Bruce reports that the animals not only have better functioning mitochondria, but they actually look and act younger. Obviously, these findings have profound implications for healthy aging.

When animal studies yield such positive and exciting results, the medical community takes notice. In the United States, cutting-edge physicians have already begun to incorporate lipoic acid in the prevention and treatment of diseases related to free radicals. As you will see, lipoic acid has already proven itself to be powerful medicine.

A cure for "incurable" mushroom poisoning

One innovative physician who has used lipoic acid in his practice for more than twenty years is Burton Berkson, M.D., Ph.D., of Las Cruces, New Mexico. Dr. Berkson can cite numerous examples of how lipoic acid has literally saved the lives of patients for whom other treatments were ineffective.

Dr. Berkson's first use of lipoic acid dates to 1977 when as a medical resident at Case Western Reserve–affiliated hospitals, he was assigned to treat a husband and wife who were suffering from liver disease caused by the highly poisonous *Amanita* mushroom. Often fatal, *Amanita* poisoning destroys the liver in several key ways, including drastically reducing the levels of glutathione, the primary antioxidant in the liver. Critically ill, the couple was expected to die within a few days.

Fortunately, Dr. Berkson knew quite a bit more about mushroom poisoning than the average physician. Before going to medical school, Dr. Berkson had earned a Ph.D. in microbiology, specializing in mycology, the study of fungi. As a mycology professor at Rutgers University, he read an article in a medical journal by a Czech doctor who described his experiences using lipoic acid as a treatment for *Amanita* poisoning. What was remarkable about the study is that out of forty patients with mushroom poisoning, thirty-nine had survived, a considerable improvement over the 60 to 90 percent mortality rate normally associated with mushroom poisoning. Dr. Berkson was eager to try lipoic acid on his two patients, but at the time, lipoic acid was available only at a handful of research centers around the world. Dr. Berkson immediately contacted Dr. Frederic Barter, who was then head of endocrinology at the National Institutes of Health in Washington, D.C., to see if anyone there was working with lipoic acid. Fortunately, Dr. Barter had some on hand, which he sent to Dr. Berkson that same day by air.

By evening, the sick couple had received their first lipoic acid treatment. To everyone's surprise, within an hour, they reported feeling markedly better. To everyone's astonishment, within three days they were getting out of bed, and within two weeks, they were back to normal. Drs. Berkson and Barter published articles on their experiences with lipoic acid in scientific journals, but few in the medical community paid any attention to them. According to Dr. Berkson, at the time the medical establishment was enamored with organ transplantation, a new and exciting field, and naively believed that the best approach to liver disease was simply to transplant a new liver.

For the past twenty years, Dr. Berkson has used lipoic acid to treat people with other forms of liver disease, such as hepatitis C, a severe infection of the liver. In fact, he notes that he has recently treated a thirty-five-year-old woman with severe hepatitis C who had been warned that she would probably die within a matter of weeks without a liver transplant. Shortly after taking lipoic acid supplements daily, she was well enough to resume her busy schedule as a working mother. Dr. Berkson's files are filled with amazing stories about "miracle cures" attributed to lipoic acid, which he describes in his new book, *Alpha Lipoic Acid: The Breakthrough Antioxidant.*

As we learn more about liver disease, there is strong evidence that lipoic acid may prove to be a useful treatment for the major cause of liver transplants in the United States, a condition called primary biliary cirrhosis (or PBC). PBC is a rare autoimmune disease of the liver that primarily affects women. In an autoimmune disease, the body's own immune cells (autoantibodies) begin to attack the body's own tissues. PBC is characterized by inflammatory destruction of hepatic bile ducts, which leads to fibrosis, cell damage, liver failure, and finally death. How can lipoic acid help? Experimental evidence has shown that these autoantibodies are directed against a specific target—the cellular proteins in the mitochondrial membrane containing lipoic acid. To me, this suggests that supplementation with lipoic acid could have a beneficial effect by interacting with these troublesome autoimmune cells before they can attack the mitochondrial proteins. In other words, lipoic acid may be able to deflect the attack before the autoimmune cells reach their target. Given the seriousness of this condition, and the recognized safety of lipoic acid, this is one area of study that should receive top priority.

Lipoic acid suppresses bad genes

I am not exaggerating when I say that one of the biggest medical stories of the century is the discovery that antioxidants play a far greater role in health maintenance than we had ever believed possible. In addition to quenching free radicals, antioxidants such as lipoic acid may prevent the onset of disease by blocking the activation of so-called bad genes. This knowledge greatly expands our ability not only to treat many different diseases, but simply to eradicate them.

There are many misconceptions about the way that genes work. For example, although most genes are normal, all of us carry a few defective or potentially harmful ones. You may believe that if you are born with a gene to develop colon cancer, heart disease, or arthritis, it automatically means that you will get that disease. That is simply not the case. Environment—lifestyle, diet, and other factors—may also play a role in determining whether we will develop a particular disease even if we are genetically programmed to do so.

Genes have to be "turned on," or activated, before they can be expressed. The body has many different signaling systems that regulate the expression of genes so that they are turned on and off at appropriate times. For example, the genes that regulate growth are more active during childhood than they are when we are fully grown adults, and that is why we stop growing at a certain point. However, if DNA is targeted by a free radical, it can activate bad genes that would have otherwise lain dormant. That is why people who are exposed to high levels of free radicals—for example, smokers—are more likely to develop particular diseases than those who are not. The free radicals in cigarette smoke may activate particular genes, which may trigger the onset of various forms of cancer and heart disease. If the person had never smoked, those genes may never have surfaced.

Hundreds of genes can also be activated by a protein called Nuclear Factor Kappa B (NF Kappa B), which can bind to DNA and alter the way it is expressed. When it is properly regulated, NF Kappa B can help the body fight against disease and perform other critical functions. If turned on too much, however, NF Kappa B can cause problems such as dampening immune function, promoting heart disease, and even accelerating skin aging.

Clearly, it is to our benefit to control NF Kappa B activation. The good news is, antioxidants in general, but lipoic acid in particular, can keep NF Kappa B contained. The bad news is, free radicals can activate NF Kappa B, which is yet another reason why it is so important to rein in free radicals before they can cause trouble.

Because antioxidants can help regulate dangerous genes, there are extraordinary possibilities to treat disease on the most basic level. If we can identify and suppress bad genes before they can do harm, we will be practicing the ultimate form of preventive medicine.

We don't have to wait to take advantage of this new information. By following the Packer Plan, we will be practicing this powerful form of preventive medicine right now.

Lipoic acid controls diabetes

Although American medicine has much to recommend it in terms of its rapid development of new drugs and lifesaving technologies, unfortunately the American medical establishment is somewhat lagging in the use of natural substances to treat common ailments. In Europe, the situation is somewhat different, and natural substances have gained a wider acceptance. The Europeans are way ahead of us in using lipoic acid as a successful treatment for a problem that is a virtual epidemic in the United States—diabetes. Before I tell you about how lipoic acid is helping diabetics by preventing some of the more severe complications associated with this disease—and how it may even help to prevent the onset of diabetes in the first place—let me tell you a bit about diabetes.

Diabetes refers to a group of biochemical disorders characterized by the body's inability to utilize carbohydrates, the sugars and starches that are found in food. In the case of diabetes, there is a snag in the metabolic machinery, which results in elevated levels of blood sugar. There is a tremendous amount of glucose in the blood, but not enough of it is getting into the cells that need it to make energy. That is why diabetes is so aptly described as "starvation amid plenty."

The two most common types are Type I diabetes, also known as juvenile (or insulin-dependent) diabetes, and Type II (or adult-onset) diabetes, also known as non-insulin-dependent diabetes mellitis (NIDDM), which accounts for about 85 percent of all cases.

Type I diabetes strikes during childhood and is caused by the failure of special cells in the pancreas called *beta cells* to produce enough insulin, the hormone that helps transport a simple sugar called glucose through the bloodstream into the muscle and fat cells. In addition to carefully controlling their diet to avoid sugar overload, Type I diabetics typically take supplemental insulin to keep their metabolic machinery functioning.

In Type II diabetes, the problem is not caused by a defect in the production of insulin; rather, it is caused by insulin resistance or impaired glucose tolerance, that is, there is plenty of insulin, but the insulin works less efficiently. In most cases, Type II diabetes can be controlled by diet and exercise; however, in some cases, medication such as insulin or drugs to lower blood sugar may also be prescribed.

Type II diabetes is a virtual epidemic in the Western world, but especially here in the United States. In fact, in our country, there are 16 million people with this form of diabetes, and probably another 50 million (one in four adults) who have a tendency to develop it under the right conditions. We know that genetics plays a part in diabetes, but apparently, so does lifestyle. People who are sedentary and overweight are much more likely to be diabetic than those who are trim and active. Type II diabetes is also more common among older people, so much so that it is considered a disease of aging. Eighty-five percent of all cases occur in people over the age of thirty-five, and with each decade, the risk of developing diabetes rises exponentially. By age seventy, you are twenty times more likely to become diabetic than you were at age fifty.

Diabetes is a serious disease that over time can cause a great deal of damage throughout the body. During the initial stages of diabetes, the microvascular system (the cells lining the blood vessels) is slightly damaged. As the disease progresses, however, the damage can become more severe, causing the blood vessels to leak, which can increase the risk of permanent nerve damage, kidney damage (nephropathy), heart disease, and blindness (retinopathy). Much of the destruction that is inflicted by this disease is either directly or indirectly caused by free radicals.

Glucose can "AGE" you

Diabetes is very much an oxidative stress disease—that is, people who are diabetic have significantly lower levels of antioxidants than normal.

This is not surprising. Oxygen loves glucose, and the bonding of the two will generate more free radicals, but that's not the only problem. Long-term exposure to glucose can also cause other serious consequences, even to nondiabetics, but especially to those who chronically suffer from elevated glucose levels.

Just as we can't live without oxygen, we can't live without glucose. If your body stops producing glucose from food, you would die of starvation because there would be no way to produce the fuel needed to run the body. Like oxygen, glucose is a dangerous friend. In a process called *glycation*, glucose reacts with proteins, such as the collagen in skin or the lenses in the eye, resulting in cross-linking of proteins. This creates a sugar-damaged protein called advanced glycation end products, or AGE for short. The acronym AGE is quite appropriate, since a high number of these damaged proteins can lead to premature aging.

The process of glycation occurs in everyone even if you are not diabetic, but there is a much higher amount of AGE in people who are diabetic. In fact, the damage to skin collagen is twice as great in diabetics as it is in nondiabetics, which is why diabetics are more vulnerable to develop brown splotches, or "age spots," on their skin, as well as premature wrinkles. In addition to inflicting cosmetic damage to skin, AGE can wreak havoc on virtually all other body tissues. For example, if the proteins in the lens of the eye become damaged, cataracts and eventual blindness may occur. If the collagen in the arteries becomes damaged, fatty plaques could form, resulting in a heart attack, or if the collagen in connective tissue becomes cross-linked, arthritis could occur. The glycation process has also been cited as a likely culprit in the destruction of nerve cells in the brain that can eventually lead to Alzheimer's and other neurodegenerative diseases. To add insult to injury, glycation can also promote the formation of free radicals. Clearly, too much glucose is not a good thing.

In order to stem the damage that can be inflicted by excess glucose, diabetes needs to be controlled as early as possible. Although lipoic acid is not a cure for diabetes, it appears to have a remarkably beneficial effect in terms of both controlling symptoms and preventing some of the serious problems that can arise down the road.

For more than twenty-five years, lipoic acid has been used in Germany to treat peripheral neuropathy caused by nerve damage at various sites of the body that can weaken muscles and cause a great deal of pain and discomfort. Peripheral nerve damage is directly related to a lack of antioxidants in nerve cells. Patients have reported a marked improvement in symptoms after being treated with high doses of lipoic acid (200 to 600 milligrams daily) either orally or intravenously, usually within two to three weeks. Dr. Stephan Jacob, M.D., of the Hypertension and Diabetes Research Center at the Max Grundig Clinic in Bühl, Germany, who has conducted several studies on the effect of lipoic acid on diabetic patients with neuropathy, told me that his patients experienced "great relief" from their symptoms, which resulted in better sleep and a general overall improvement. In addition, his patients reported feeling more fit and better able to keep up with their work. Several also noted that they were able to reduce their doses of insulin or anti-diabetic pills. After taking lipoic acid, they not only felt better, they felt healthier.

Recently, Dr. Dan Ziegler and Dr. F. Arnold Gries at Heinrich Heine University in Düsseldorf had even more exciting news to report about lipoic acid. They found that treatment with lipoic acid actually stimulated the regeneration of nerve fibers in diabetics. In as little as three weeks of treatment, patients taking 600 milligrams of lipoic acid daily experienced a significant reduction in pain and numbness associated with neuropathy.

In addition to boosting the body's levels of antioxidants, lipoic acid works to control diabetes in several other noteworthy ways, including by reducing protein damage (AGE) in animals and humans. Since the formation of AGE is not just a problem for diabetics but is a factor in the aging process itself, here is good evidence that lipoic acid may help to slow down aging in general. Since lipoic acid can help improve the utilization of glucose by muscle cells, it is highly likely that lipoic acid supplements may help prevent the onset of Type II diabetes in the first place.

Positive reports on lipoic acid have attracted the attention of Dr. Peter Dyck and Dr. Phillip A. Low of the Mayo Clinic and Foundation, who are planning a multicenter trial investigating lipoic acid as a treatment for diabetic polyneuropathy. I suspect that the results in the U.S. study will be as good as those achieved in Europe.

I am not suggesting that diabetics should self-medicate with lipoic acid—diabetes is a disease that needs to be carefully managed by a skilled physician. I do believe, however, that lipoic acid can be incorporated into the treatment of diabetes along with other therapies. Since most physicians are unfamilar with lipoic acid, I have included an extensive bibliography citing pertinent studies that can help physicians learn how to incorporate lipoic acid into the treatment regimen of their diabetic patients.

Lipoic acid, AIDS, and immune function

Disease and oxidative stress are closely linked: even a disease that appears to be totally unrelated to the body's tug-of-war between free radicals and antioxidants can be profoundly affected by a shift in the antioxidant balance. Such is the case with AIDS (acquired immune deficiency syndrome), which is actually a group of diseases that result from the suppression of the immune system by the human immuno-deficiency virus (HIV). A retrovirus is a virus that can alter the genetic makeup of a cell. What makes HIV so difficult to control is that this virus targets and destroys immune cells called *T-helper cells,* the body's first line of defense against infection. Once the T-cells are decimated, the body is left vulnerable to a host of opportunistic infections that prey on weakened immune systems. For example, people with AIDS are especially vulnerable to pneumonia and cytomegalovirus (which can cause blindness), two infections that a healthy immune system can often defeat.

Although AIDS appears to be caused solely by an infectious agent, the reality is that oxidative stress is a major factor in the progression of the virus. When the T-cells are weakened by HIV, they lose their ability to produce and transport glutathione, a major cellular antioxidant. Once the T-cells lose their antioxidant edge, they succumb to oxidative stress, which can cause even further destruction. Not surprisingly, the glutathione levels as well as levels of other antioxidants are significantly lower in HIV-positive patients. Although restoring antioxidants is not a cure for AIDS, researchers believe that it, along with other medications, will at least help give the body a fighting chance against the virus.

In the test tube, lipoic acid prevents the replication of HIV in cultured human cells. Although this doesn't necessarily mean that it will work in HIV-positive people, I think it might. There is also some evidence that lipoic acid bolsters the antioxidant defenses in HIV-positive people, which presumably will help them fight infections better. In one study, lipoic acid (150 milligrams three times daily) was given orally to twelve HIV-positive patients. At the end of the two weeks, all of the patients had an increase in blood glutathione levels, and nine of the patients had an increase in the number of T-helper cells—a sign that their immune systems were stronger. More studies are needed to determine if lipoic acid should be included in the treatment of HIV infection, but it seems obvious that restoring the antioxidant balance can help. If you are HIV-positive, I recommend that you find a knowledgeable physician who can help determine if lipoic acid supplements should be added to your treatment regimen.

Lipoic acid is a memory enhancer

As we age, there is a subtle but very real decline in mental function that begins during midlife. The most common symptom is the deterioration of short-term memory, known as age-associated memory impairment (AAMI). A name forgotten, a missed appointment, even the loss of mental stamina are all signs of AAMI. I want to stress that these temporary lapses are not signs of senility or Alzheimer's disease; they are a normal part of the aging process. The good news is, antioxidants may play a role in helping to preserve mental function.

Brain cells, or *neurons,* communicate with one another by releasing chemicals called *neurotransmitters.* As we age, there is a significant decline in production of neurotransmitters, as well as the loss of brain cells, which may contribute to so-called brain aging. Other factors also come into play.

As the regulator of all body functions, the brain is one of our hardest working organs. In fact, it is a virtual hotbed of activity, and it requires a tremendous amount of energy to carry on its work. This 1-pound organ coordinates all of the body's nervous activity, processes incoming sensory impulses, and is the repository of reasoning, intellect, memory, consciousness, and emotions. As a result, the brain consumes a vast amount of energy. To accommodate its insatiable need for energy, brain tissue is rich in mitochondria, the cellular powerhouses that produce ATP, the fuel that runs the body. Since the burning of oxygen is required to make energy, the brain is also a major producer of free radicals and is particularly vulnerable to oxidative stress. Over time, the constant assault of free radicals can exact a steep toll on mental function.

Since free radical damage has been implicated in age-related changes in memory, researchers have investigated whether supplemental antioxidants can help slow down this damage—and perhaps even reverse it.

A recent study performed at the Clinical Institute for Mental Health in Mannheim, Germany, examined the effect of lipoic acid on memory loss in aging mice, which experience similar age-related memory problems as humans. Older but otherwise healthy mice were given lipoic acid in their drinking water. After fourteen days of treatment, the mice had to negotiate their way through a maze. Mice treated with lipoic acid performed significantly better than untreated mice. Many did as well and some even better than mice half their age. The researchers speculated that by boosting antioxidant levels, lipoic acid reduced the amount of oxidative stress in the brain, or perhaps it even slowed down the age-related loss of brain cells. Interestingly, lipoic acid did not improve performance in younger animals that presumably still have strong antioxidant defenses.

More studies are required to determine whether lipoic acid will enhance mental function in humans, but there is strong evidence that many antioxidants (specifically vitamin E, ginkgo biloba, and the pine bark extract supplement Pycnogenol) certainly can play a role in keeping us smart and sharp at any age.

Lipoic acid and radiation poisoning

Exposure to radiation produces a cascade of free radicals that causes severe damage and can be fatal. Radiation decimates the body's supply of glutathione, which allows free radicals to severely damage the body's tissues and organs. Several antioxidant compounds have been used to treat radiation damage, with varying degrees of effectiveness. In fact, virtually every army in the world equips its soldiers with antiradiation drugs that are similar in molecular structure to two antioxidants— glutathione and lipoic acid. Recently, researchers at the Russian Institute of Pediatric Hematology and the Vitamin Research Institute in Moscow have found that lipoic acid may prove to be one of most effective antiradiation treatments to date.

Radiation is so deadly that when animals are exposed to high levels of radiation, only 35 percent of them will survive. Lipoic acid is so powerful that if the animals are treated with lipoic acid before exposure, the survival rate increases to 90 percent. Although we don't know precisely why more mice survive, I suspect it is because of lipoic acid's ability to boost the immune system, enhancing the body's ability to fight against diseases generated by free radicals.

Fortunately, most of us have never been exposed to lethal levels of radiation, but accidents do happen. The near meltdown of a nuclear power plant in Chernobyl, Ukraine, in 1986 led to radioactive fallout and massive soil contamination in the surrounding area. People who continued to live in Chernobyl were exposed to constant low levels of radiation. As a result, the incidence of cancer is much higher than normal, particularly among children.

Researchers examined the effects of lipoic acid treatment on the level of oxidative damage in children living in areas affected by the Chernobyl accident. The higher the level of blood peroxidation, the greater the sign of damage caused by free radicals. After twenty-eight days of lipoic acid supplements, researchers had some extraordinarily good news to report. They found that in children treated with lipoic acid, blood peroxidation levels had fallen to those seen in normal children. Even better, the children's liver and kidney functions were normalized. Even against the powerful free radicals generated by radiation exposure, lipoic acid was able to hold its own.

Lipoic acid: the smoker's rescue formula

I am delighted to report that along with three colleagues—Gladys Block, Ph.D.; Maret Traber, Ph.D.; and Carol Cross, M.D.—I have recently undertaken a unique clinical study that could ultimately benefit the tens of millions of Americans who smoke.

Before I begin, let me make my position on smoking perfectly clear. If you smoke, quitting smoking is the single most important thing you can do to safeguard your health and ultimately save your life. Smoking is a leading cause of death in the Western world, and on average, it will rob you of about eight years of life. I think most smokers know these dismal facts, and that is why out of the 40 million smokers in the United States, at any given time 30 million would like to quit. Unfortunately, smoking is a highly addictive habit, and quitting is very difficult, so difficult in fact that 90 percent of those who give up smoking start smoking again within five years. Until people do stop smoking, they can try to protect their health the best way they can.

Here are the facts: Smokers have elevated risks of developing heart disease, diabetes, stroke, and some forms of cancer, and to a lesser extent, so do people who are exposed to secondhand smoke. There is no doubt that oxidative stress contributes to the onset and progression of these diseases. Each puff of cigarette smoke contains thousands of different free radicals that can overwhelm the body's antioxidant defenses. Smokers have lower plasma levels of vitamins E and C and glutathione. I think that it is obvious that the constant drain on the body's antioxidant system puts smokers at great risk of disease.

I believe that it may be possible to reduce the risk of disease associated with cigarette smoke by bolstering the network antioxidants with supplements. There have been attempts to reduce the risk of smoking by giving smokers beta carotene (which is not a network antioxidant), and as I explain in the chapter on carotenoids, these experiments failed miserably. There have also been studies in which smokers have been given vitamins C and E, which appeared to reduce their levels of oxidative stess. But, to date, there has never been a study designed specifically to boost the entire antioxidant network in general, and glutathione in particular. By the time this book goes to press, my laboratory will be undertaking a study to determine whether an antioxidant cocktail (spelled out in Part Four) can help boost antioxidant levels in smokers, and whether it will reduce oxidative stress and disease.

In our study, we will be recruiting 500 subjects from the Kaiser Foundation in Oakland, California. This group will include smokers, nonsmokers, and passive smokers—people who live or work with smokers but do not smoke themselves. From this study, we hope to learn whether the antioxidant cocktail will reduce oxidative stress injury in both smokers and passive smokers. This would be the first step in determining whether the antioxidant network can actually protect smokers against the free radical damage inflicted by cigarette smoke.

It could be years before we publish our results, and many smokers may want to know if they should begin the antioxidant cocktail right now. My answer is a strong yes. I feel that boosting the antioxidant network will prove to have a positive effect on the health of smokers and, next to quitting, is an important way you can protect your body from some of the damage inflicted by cigarette smoke.

As important as lipoic acid may be in the antioxidant network, it is just one part of an exciting, ongoing story that continues to unfold daily. I believe that we have barely scratched the surface in terms of fully understanding the power of this antioxidant and how to use it to its full potential.

5

Vitamin E

An Extraordinary Antioxidant

An antiaging antioxidant, vitamin E, reverses the age-related "slump" in immune function and keeps your brain cells from aging. It works better than a prescription drug in delaying the onset of Alzheimer's disease.

Taking vitamin E supplements daily will substantially reduce your risk of heart attack and stroke. If you've already had a heart attack, vitamin E can significantly reduce your risk of having a second one.

* Vitamin E keeps your skin youthful by protecting against damage from UV radiation and ozone, the major causes of wrinkles, brown spots, and even cancer.

* Vitamin E relieves symptoms of arthritis and other inflammatory diseases.

* Vitamin E reduces the risk of prostate cancer in men and can inhibit the growth of breast cancer cells.

* *RDA:* 30 I.U.

❋ *The Packer Plan:* 500 milligrams daily of mixed tocopherols and tocotrienols.

❋ *Sources:* Raw vegetable oils, nuts, nut butters, rice bran oil, barley, and in smaller amounts in green leafy vegetables.

"I take vitamin E for my heart."

"I started taking vitamin E after I read in a health magazine that it was good for arthritis. It's helped a lot."

"I take vitamin E to keep me looking young."

If you asked a roomful of people why they take vitamin E—as we recently did—you are bound to get dozens of different answers. When it comes to vitamin E, everyone has his or her own opinion.

For more than seventy years, vitamin E has been the subject of intense scrutiny, debate, and speculation. Before we even knew what vitamin E did, opponents dismissed it as worthless, and its supporters claimed that it was a virtual cure-all for everything from arthritis to infertility to cancer.

Many decades and thousands of studies later, the news about vitamin E is nothing short of breathtaking, and even its most ardent supporters could not have imagined the breadth and scope of its potential benefits.

I have been studying vitamin E for more than thirty years and have been involved in much of the scientific research that has led to breakthroughs in our understanding of this vitamin. In fact, the Packer Lab is located in the same building at the University of California at Berkeley where the two scientists who first discovered vitamin E did some of their most exciting and creative work.

Before I tell you about its spectacular present, let me review some of vitamin E's intriguing past. Vitamin E was identified in 1922 by scientists Herbert Evans and Katherine Bishop, who observed that an unidentified substance found in green lettuce prevented rats from miscarrying. If the rats were not fed green lettuce, they could not carry to term. This mysterious substance was finally isolated from wheat germ oil in 1936, also at Berkeley, and named *tocopherol* from the Greek words *tokos* (childbirth) and *pherein* (to carry). The *-ol* suffix signifies that the compound is a *phenol* or alcohol. Because vitamin E could prevent miscarriage in rats, it quickly became known among the public as the vitamin that could make you "sexy," which of course made serious scientists extremely wary of it.

Vitamin E is a family of molecules composed of four different tocopherols and four different tocotrienols, all nearly identical in structure. Although alpha tocopherol is the best-known family member, its other siblings are also extremely important. Unfortunately, modern food processing routinely depletes our food supply of all forms of natural vitamin E, which leaves many of us deficient in this key antioxidant. About half of all U.S. adults take vitamin E supplements, but most vitamin E supplements contain only one kind of vitamin E—alpha tocopherol—but not the others. If you are just taking alpha tocopherol, you are missing out on the full range of benefits offered by the entire vitamin E family. That is why I recommend taking a vitamin E supplement that includes the entire spectrum of all the natural vitamin Es, tocopherols *and* tocotrienols.

Other than preventing miscarriage in rodents, vitamin E's role in the body eluded researchers. Animal studies showed that extreme vitamin E deficiencies caused wasting and severe muscle weakness. Biochemists knew that vitamin E was an antioxidant and could prevent the oxidative damage that caused polyunsaturated fats and oils to become rancid when exposed to air. In fact, an early commercial use of vitamin E was to retard food spoilage. But this did not seem relevant to human beings because, at that time, there was no evidence that fats were actually oxidized in the body.

In a groundbreaking experiment in 1954, A. L. Tappel, a renowned biochemist at the University of California at Davis, finally proved that in the same manner in which vitamin E prevented the fat in food from going rancid from oxidation, it also prevented the fat in our blood from going rancid from the same enemy—oxygen. The oxidation of fat in the body is known as lipid peroxidation and is now believed to be the underlying cause of heart disease. More important, Dr. Tappel showed that vitamin E could stop lipid peroxidation dead in its tracks.

I first met Dr. Tappel in 1959 when I was a postgraduate student at the University of Pennsylvania and he was a visiting professor looking for a laboratory to set up shop. Much to my delight, he chose mine, and by doing so kindled my interest in vitamin E. Al Tappel and I are an unlikely pair. He is as quiet and unassuming as I am talkative and outgoing. In the laboratory, he is almost militarylike in his execution of plans and works with an intensity that belies his otherwise easygoing personality. Yet we forged a wonderful working relationship that developed into a lifelong friendship. At the University of Pennsylvania, after a long day at work, we would walk home through the streets of West Philadelphia, speculating about what impact our research on antioxidants would eventually have on science in general and the practice of medicine in particular. I am delighted to note that many of the things we predicted back then have come to pass. We later became colleagues when I joined the faculty of the University of California.

Much of my work has focused on vitamin E's role in the antioxidant network, where it functions as the body's primary fat-soluble antioxidant.

In the antioxidant network, vitamin E is recycled by vitamin C, lipoic acid, and Coenzyme Q10. Even if you take vitamin C and lipoic acid, you still need to take vitamin E. Each network antioxidant has its own job to perform that cannot be duplicated by the others.

What makes vitamin E unique is that it can maneuver through the fatty parts of the cell membrane, which are inaccessible to the other network antioxidants. Only vitamin E can move in this medium, targeting and quenching free radicals in the process. Since vitamin E is soluble in fat, and not in blood, which is primarily water, in order to travel through the bloodstream, vitamin E must be carried in a complex particle called a lipoprotein, which is produced in the liver and travels through the blood, delivering fat and cholesterol to cells for growth and maintenance.

There are several kinds of lipoproteins, depending on the types of fat they transport. Low-density lipoprotein (LDL), also known as bad cholesterol, delivers cholesterol to the tissues. High-density lipoprotein (HDL), also known as good cholesterol, carries cholesterol back to the liver to be excreted in the bile.

Compared to the number of fat molecules in cell membranes, vitamin E is present in astonishingly low concentrations—for every 1,000 to 2,000 lipid molecules, there is only 1 molecule of vitamin E. Even though vitamin E is present in such minuscule amounts, it performs a vital job. Practically single-handedly, vitamin E protects lipoproteins from free radical damage, or oxidation, the same process that turns butter rancid. Vitamin E is often called a "chain-breaking" antioxidant because it halts the biochemical chain of events that leads to the spread of free radicals, which can seriously damage lipids and proteins.

High levels of lipoproteins are a risk factor for heart disease, as well as many other diseases, including cancer. In fact, you have undoubtedly heard that a higher than normal cholesterol level can significantly increase your risk of having a heart attack. A high cholesterol level is an indication that your body is not processing lipoproteins rapidly enough, which means that lipoproteins are lingering in your bloodstream. This in turn increases the risk of free radical attack, which can initiate a cascade of events that eventually lead to heart disease.

Vitamin E is a cancer fighter

Free radical attack of lipids and proteins can also damage DNA, the genetic material within the cell, which can lead to cancer.

Quenching free radicals is not the only way vitamin E can help keep cancer at bay. Each of the network antioxidants in general, and vitamin E in particular, appears to play a much greater role in regulating body systems than was ever believed possible. As is lipoic acid, vitamin E is involved in signaling pathways that turn on and off genes and regulate cell growth. In particular, researchers such as my friend and colleague Angelo Azzi, in Bern, Switzerland, have found that vitamin E inhibits protein kinase C activity, which activates enzymes that stimulate tumor growth. Numerous studies confirm that people who eat a diet rich in vitamin E and other antioxidants have significantly lower rates of cancer than those who don't. Other studies have linked low levels of vitamin E to an increased risk of many different kinds of cancer, but especially prostate and lung cancer. In fact, Katalin G. Losonczy, a researcher with the National Institute on Aging, studied the consumption of vitamin E among 11,798 people ages 65 to 105. She found that those who took vitamin E supplements daily were 41 percent less likely to have died from cancer, and 40 percent less likely to have died from heart disease, than people who didn't take vitamin E.

Vitamin E and longevity

Studies such as the one that I have just described beg the question about whether people who take vitamin E will live longer than those who don't. There is no simple answer to this question, but all signs point to a resounding *yes*. Even better, antioxidants such as vitamin E can enhance the *quality* of life in those later years and set the stage for healthy aging.

In studies of human cells, we have wonderful evidence that vitamin E can prevent aging on the cellular level, which is where the aging process begins. Long before we can see the outward manifestations of aging, such as wrinkles and gray hair, subtle changes are occurring to our cells. One of the telltale signs of aging is the accumulation of an age pigment called *lipofuscin* in all the specialized cells of the body, but especially in the brain and heart. Lipofuscin is a direct result of lipid peroxidation, or the oxidation of proteins and lipids. In other words, our cells become rancid.

My colleague David Deamer, Ph.D., at the University of California at Davis performed an experiment that dramatically shows the effect of vitamin E on cellular aging. He grew young cells in a culture of 10 percent serum in which they grew normally and did not show signs of lipofuscin until they reached a ripe old age. He then grew the same type of cells in a low serum medium in which they were nutrient-deprived and could not divide or repair themselves as needed. Under these conditions, they accumulated a huge amount of age pigment early in their life span, a sign of premature aging. If you look at these cells under a fluorescent microscope, you can clearly see a mass of yellow that you do not see in normal young cells, indicating a high amount of lipofuscin. However, when Dr. Deamer grew the same cells in a nutrient-deprived environment but added 100 micrograms of vitamin E, they did not develop lipofuscin. The cells remained "young."

Maintaining cellular health is the key to preventing the diseases of aging, and that is the key to promoting longevity. Vitamin E is a powerful antioxidant that can help us maintain our antioxidant advantage and ward off the diseases that cut life short.

Reducing the oxidative stress on our bodies may indeed have a profound effect on extending our lives. In one intriguing experiment performed at my laboratory more than twenty-five years ago, we found that in culture, vitamin E was actually able to extend the life of a common type of human cell. There are hundreds of different human cell types. Some are unique to particular organ systems—for example, the cardiac muscle has specialized cells called *cardiac myocytes* and the liver has cells called *hepatocytes*. What all human cells have in common is a designated life span. Each cell in the body is programmed to divide a certain number of times before it dies. Scientists believe that there is actually a "clock" within each cell that regulates the number of cell divisions. This is known as the *Hayflick phenomenon,* in honor of the scientist who first made this observation. There have been several fascinating studies in which cells have been frozen—which in effect stops the cellular clock—but when they are thawed, they pick up where they left off and continue to divide on schedule.

There are a number of different factors that can affect the life of a cell, including illness and the number of times it must divide to repair itself. The more demands placed on a cell—that is, the more frequently it must divide—the shorter its life.

In our study, we grew a cell type identified as WI 38 embryonic human lung cell, which is reported to have a limited life span of about fifty divisions when grown in a culture outside of the body. Our objective was to determine whether adding vitamin E to the cell culture would affect the length of time it stayed viable. In one series of experiments, vitamin E actually *doubled* the life span of the cells. Instead of dividing the usual 50 times, the cells amazingly divided more than 100 times. Similar studies have been reported in other laboratories. It is very likely that reducing oxidative stress—that is, fortifying the cells with additional antioxidant protection—was responsible for extending their lives.

In another experiment, we further proved the power of vitamin E in protecting against oxidative stress by "stressing out" human cells. When we exposed human cells to visible light at their twenty-fifth doubling (roughly middle age), they died rapidly because the light initiated the formation of free radicals that damaged these cells. When we pretreated the cells with high levels of vitamin E before exposure to light, miraculously they all survived and lived out their normal life span.

At the time that I published the results of these experiments in the *Proceedings of the National Academy of Sciences,* I noted: "We interpret this result as support for the free radical theory of aging." Simply put, taking antioxidants will help us live longer. These and other similar studies merely confirm the wisdom of maintaining the antioxidant advantage.

Vitamin E and heart disease

Vitamin E's powerful protection against heart disease is a prime example of the Antioxidant Miracle in action. There is overwhelming evidence that vitamin E decreases the risk of developing heart disease and can even prevent a second heart attack in patients who already have heart disease.

The term "heart disease" most often refers to coronary artery disease, a condition that occurs when the arteries feeding blood to the heart become narrowed or blocked entirely. Although deaths from heart disease have been steadily declining since the second half of this century, it is still the leading cause of death in the Western world. We now understand more about heart disease than ever before, and I like to think that we cell biologists have played a pivotal role in helping to unravel this mystery. Certainly, those of us who have studied vitamin E and other antioxidants can take pride that we may have helped save some lives.

As far back as 1933, Wilfred Shute and Evan Shute, two cardiologists in London, Ontario, Canada, began using vitamin E to treat heart conditions. In their 1972 book, *Vitamin E for Healthy and Ailing Hearts,* the Shutes reported having treated more than 30,000 patients with vitamin E, with overwhelmingly positive results. In fact, the Shutes suggested the then-radical concept that by taking vitamin E and making other changes in diet and lifestyle, people could prevent suffering from heart disease in the first place. Although the public embraced their message, and vitamin E became a popular supplement, the initial reaction of the medical community was to dismiss their claims as ridiculous and the Shutes as misguided at best, and hucksters at worst. The notion that a simple vitamin pill could have a profound effect on the health and well-being of patients was considered absurd. Back then, preventive medicine wasn't even given lip service, much less practiced.

The medical community was still mesmerized by expensive, complicated approaches to health care—the more costly and high-tech the better. Spectacular medical advancements such as the angiogram, which for the first time provided an accurate image of the heart, and the heart-lung machine, which took over for the patient's heart during surgery, made open heart surgery a reality. In fact, coronary bypass surgery (in which the blocked artery was replaced by a vein taken from another part of the body) was the treatment of choice for coronary artery disease. Undoubtedly, many lives were saved by coronary bypass surgery, but as the number of surgeries began to skyrocket, many people began to wonder if too many surgeons were jumping the gun and opting for surgery before trying noninvasive treatments first.

By the early 1980s, there were close to 200,000 coronary bypass surgeries performed annually. And far from being a permanent cure for heart disease, doctors were finding that within a short time, the arteries of bypass patients filled up again with plaque, and the surgery had to be redone. Prosurgery attitudes quickly changed as the results of several well-publicized studies raised doubts about whether bypass patients showed any improvement in longevity or recurrence of heart attack compared with those who were treated with medication. At the same time, a growing body of scientific research began to unravel the causes of heart disease, and it became impossible to ignore the role of diet in general, and antioxidants in particular, in the onset and progression of this disease.

Much of the work performed on vitamin E in my laboratory and others like it provided the model for establishing its role in the prevention of heart disease. Our work provided the molecular explanation for the phenomenal results that physicians such as the Shutes and researchers were reporting in animal and human studies.

Although many people are often taken by surprise by a heart attack or the onset of angina (chest pain), in reality the disease has been developing silently over decades before it produces any symptoms.

Heart disease begins when LDL invades the lining of the capillary/coronary wall and becomes oxidized. Under ideal conditions, the vitamin E in the LDL will trap the free radical and destroy it. In the process, the vitamin E becomes a weak free radical itself. If the antioxidant network is working well, vitamin C or lipoic acid will then recharge the vitamin E, turning it back into an antioxidant. However, if the network is overwhelmed—that is, if the body is under a great deal of oxidative stress—the vitamin E will not be recycled, and the lipoprotein will be defenseless against free radical attack. Lipids and proteins will suffer oxidative damage, triggering the formation of plaque, which can clog arteries. As the plaque deposits grow, key arteries can become narrowed, compromising the flow of blood to the heart.

The ultimate cause of heart disease is a failure of the body's antioxidant network to do its job. Bolstering vitamin E and the entire antioxidant network will have a profound effect on our ability to fight heart disease.

Two famous Harvard-based population studies involving both men and women health-care professionals prove this point. In one follow-up study of more than 87,000 women nurses, those who took vitamin E supplements for more than two years had a 41 percent lower risk of developing major heart disease than those who did not. In another study of close to 29,000 male health professionals, those who consumed at least 200 I.U. daily of vitamin E had a 37 percent lower risk of heart disease than those not taking vitamin E. I hasten to point out that based on these studies, we can conclude that many physicians are taking vitamin E, even though they may not admit it to their patients!

If you're not convinced yet that you should be taking vitamin E, consider the following studies:

* Doctors Ishwarlal Jialal and Sridevi Devaraj of the University of Texas Southwestern Medical Center studied the effect of 1,200 I.U. of vitamin E on the level of oxidized LDL in twenty-one healthy subjects. At the end of eight weeks, the susceptibility of LDL to become oxidized decreased an average of 40 percent. They also saw a decrease in the amount of free radicals released by monocytes, white cells that gobble up oxidized LDL and initiate the atherosclerotic process. Here was evidence that vitamin E stopped the onset of heart disease at its earliest stage. More important, Dr. Jialal found that it takes a *minimum* of 400 I.U. of vitamin E daily to protect LDL from oxidation.

* In another study published in 1996, researchers examined the degree of blockage in coronary arteries. They found a remarkable inverse correlation between the severity of the disease and the amount of vitamin E in LDL. Patients with the highest content of E in their LDL had the lowest degree of blockage; patients with the lowest content of E in their LDL had the highest degree of blockage.

Clearly, the amount of vitamin E in LDL can make a profound difference in terms of developing heart disease, and how fast the disease progresses.

It's never too late for vitamin E

The good news is, even if you have heart disease, it's not too late to benefit from vitamin E. The most dramatic study to date attesting to the benefits of vitamin E was performed on patients who had already been diagnosed with one heart attack. The Cambridge Heart Antioxidant Study (known as CHAOS) was a double-blind, placebo-controlled study of 2,002 people with diagnosed heart disease, 37 percent of whom were in very serious condition or had already had triple bypass surgery. Some

1,035 patients were given either 400 I.U. or 800 I.U. of vitamin E daily. The remaining 967 received a placebo. Within 510 days, researchers found that the patients who had been taking vitamin E had an amazing 77 percent fewer heart attacks than those who didn't. Given the results of this study, which was published in the British medical journal *Lancet,* researchers decided to discontinue the study and prescribe vitamin E to all of the patients. What is particularly noteworthy about this study is that it shows that vitamin E can protect the hearts of even the highest-risk people.

There are a growing number of physicians who prescribe vitamin E to their patients to prevent or treat heart disease. Julian Whitaker, M.D., of the Whitaker Wellness Institute in Newport Beach, California, a leading proponent of vitamin E therapy for heart patients, told me, "I've been using vitamin E in my practice for more than two decades. Based on the experiences of thousands of patients, I can say unequivocally that supplementing with vitamin E daily is more powerful in the treatment of heart disease than making dietary changes."

I believe that vitamin E, along with the entire antioxidant network, can save countless more lives by preventing the internal environment that gives rise to heart disease in the first place. To me, this is a far more intelligent approach than trying to correct the problem after the fact.

The neglected vitamin E family members

When it comes to vitamin E, the liver plays favorites; it contains a protein that sorts out the various forms of tocopherols and tocotrienols, and primarily selects alpha tocopherol to insert into the lipoproteins. Why the liver prefers alpha tocopherol is somewhat of a mystery and may not be in our best interest. The mechanism that conserves alpha tocopherol is probably inherited from preindustrial times when alpha tocopherol was very scarce in the diet. Because the body favors alpha tocopherol, many scientists have focused on this form of vitamin E to the exclusion of its two important cousins, tocotrienols and gamma tocopherol. Recently, however, researchers have uncovered some fascinating new information about these neglected members of the vitamin E family.

Tocotrienols: the bodyguards

Tocotrienols are the form of vitamin E found in cereal brans, such as rice bran, wheat bran, and oat bran. Tocotrienols have the same basic functions as tocopherols but at the molecular level have a different shape, which gives them some special powers above their antioxidant function.

These members of the vitamin E family have a unique role in helping to prevent and to treat conditions such as atherosclerosis (clogged arteries), high cholesterol levels, and even some cancers.

Stroke is one of the life-threatening conditions that might be prevented and treated by tocotrienols. A stroke is usually caused by a narrowing of the carotid artery in the neck caused by plaque deposits, which cuts off the blood supply to the brain. Patients diagnosed with carotid stenosis (a narrowing of the carotid artery) are at high risk of stroke. Until now, the only treatment for carotid stenosis was a dangerous surgical procedure known as carotid endarterectomy in which the arteries are cut open and scraped clean. What makes this procedure so risky is the possibility that a piece of debris will travel upstream to the brain, thereby causing a stroke, the very condition it was meant to prevent.

The good news is that tocotrienols may be a safe alternative to surgery for patients with carotid stenosis. In a four-year study, patients with severe carotid stenosis were given either tocotrienols or a placebo. Each patient's progress was measured by an ultrasound examination, which produces a picture of the carotid artery. Ultrasound scans of the patients were performed at six months, twelve months, and yearly thereafter.

The results were quite remarkable: 94 percent of the patients receiving tocotrienols improved or stabilized, whereas none of the controls improved, and over half got worse. What is particularly noteworthy about this study is that it is the first study to produce a regression in clogged arteries and an improvement in arterial health and blood flow in humans.

The incredible improvement in the group receiving tocotrienols was evident after six months and has been maintained ever since, whereas the placebo group has continued to deteriorate.

The cardiologist, Dr. Marvin Bierenbaum of the Kenneth L. Jordan Heart Foundation in Montclair, New Jersey, who conducted the study noted, "The results are a breakthrough. We think that the alpha tocopherol is protecting LDL from oxidation and that the tocotrienols are cleaning up the arterial walls. There are hundreds of thousands of North Americans diagnosed with carotid stenosis. Up until now, their choices have been dismal. Basically, we used to monitor them until the arterial blockage got so bad that there was no choice but complex, high-tech, high-risk surgery. For these patients, tocotrienols are an alternative to surgery."

Dr. Bierenbaum notes that for the 50 million U.S. men and women with high blood pressure who are at an increased risk of having a stroke, supplementation with tocotrienols may help arterial blockages from developing in the first place.

That's not all tocotrienols can do. Dr. Bierenbaum discovered that rice-bran tocotrienols contain phytochemicals that enhance the cholesterol-lowering effect of tocotrienols. After three years, Dr. Bierenbaum switched the patients from palm-derived tocotrienols to 400 milligrams of rice-bran tocotrienols. The same patients whose cholesterol levels had remained unmodified by palm tocotrienols experienced dramatic reductions in LDL (the so-called "bad" cholesterol) and a 20 percent increase in HDL ("good" cholesterol) when switched to rice tocotrienols. More important, the total cholesterol-to-HDL ratio improved by 28 percent, which sharply reduces the risk of dying from heart disease. These natural antioxidants extracted from rice bran outperformed most of the lipid-lowering drugs, and are a promising alternative to statin drugs.

Other studies have shown that tocotrienols reduce blood glucose levels, protect against liver disease, and reduce the levels of thromboxane A2, a clotting factor that increases the risk for strokes and heart attacks.

Recently, we have learned that tocotrienols may be a powerful weapon against breast cancer. There are two types of breast cancer: estrogen-positive and estrogen-negative. Estrogen-positive cancers are estrogen-sensitive, which means that estrogen can stimulate the tumors to grow. Estrogen-negative cancers are not affected by estrogen. Younger women tend to develop estrogen-negative cancers, while postmenopausal women typically have estrogen-positive cancers. The antiestrogen drug tamoxifen has been used successfully in both the prevention and treatment of estrogen-positive cancer, but it is not effective against estrogen-negative cancer. Tamoxifen can also produce devastating side effects including uterine cancer. Researchers from the University of Western

Ontario published a study comparing the effect of tamoxifen and tocotrienols on both estrogen-positive and estrogen-negative breast cancer cells. In the test tube, tocotrienols inhibited the growth of *both* kinds of breast cancer cells. In fact, tocotrienols worked so well that researchers are investigating the possibility of incorporating them in breast cancer therapy along with drugs such as tamoxifen, which are also given to prevent breast cancer in high-risk women. I believe that clinical trials testing the effect of tocotrienols on breast cancer patients, combined with other network antioxidants such as Co Q10 and lipoic acid, are urgently needed.

What makes tocotrienols so special? I believe the explanation for these important effects lies in the special way that tocotrienols maneuver around the cell membrane and the relative ease with which tocotrienols interact with other elements in the antioxidant network. At the Packer Lab, we have shown that tocotrienols are mobile and distribute evenly through biological membranes, whereas tocopherols tend to cluster in islands. In other words, they can get into tight spots that the tocopherols cannot. To add to their unique abilities, tocotrienols are forty to sixty times more readily recycled than tocopherols, which means that they have more staying power.

Work in the Packer Lab has revealed another secret about tocotrienols—the skin loves them. We found that ingested tocotrienols are readily taken up by cells in the skin, which suggests to me that they may have an important function against the aging effects of ultraviolet light and ozone. Last year, Maret Traber, one of the world's leading vitamin E researchers, and I presented this work to an international conference in Penang, Malaysia.

Tocotrienols are important constituents of the antioxidant network because they are mobile within membranes and are readily recycled by other members of the antioxidant network.

Tocotrienols are doubly blessed: They keep your arteries young on the inside and your skin young on the outside!

Gamma tocopherol: the smoker's friend

Gamma tocopherol is the natural form of vitamin E present in soy and corn oils. Unfortunately, most of the gamma tocopherol is gone from these oils before they reach the consumer, which means that our diets are deficient in this form of vitamin E. The gamma tocopherol–rich fraction is stripped off during refining and sold separately to vitamin E manufacturers, which, in turn, convert it to alpha tocopherol and sell it as natural vitamin E. As a result, food products such as shortenings, salad dressings, and baked foods that used to contain natural gamma tocopherol in abundance are now manufactured from refined oils that have been largely stripped of vitamin E. Manufacturers often add cheaper synthetic alpha tocopherol to processed foods so that products such as potato chips, which used to be a rich dietary source of gamma tocopherol, now contain almost exclusively synthetic alpha tocopherol.

Whereas thirty years ago, natural gamma tocopherol was the dominant form of vitamin E in the North American diet, the use of synthetic alpha tocopherol and the extraction of gamma tocopherol from food oils to manufacture natural alpha tocopherol have shifted the balance.

Ironically, now that we have depleted the food supply of gamma tocopherol, recent research is pointing to a significant role in the body for gamma tocopherol. In particular, gamma tocopherol may help to block the biochemical pathways that trigger inflammation as well as cancer.

Studies have shown that the ratio of gamma tocopherol to alpha tocopherol in serum is depressed in patients who smoke cigarettes, have cardiovascular disease, or are suffering from AIDS. This deficiency could be significant in terms of hampering the body's ability to fight against the inflammation that can aggravate these problems.

For smokers, a deficiency in gamma tocopherol could be deadly. A population study compared the residents of the Cook Islands and the Fiji Islands in the South Pacific. There are similar patterns of smoking in both populations. However, the serum gamma tocopherol levels are twice as high in the Fijians as compared with the Cook Islanders whereas alpha tocopherol levels are the same. The incidence of lung cancer in Fijians is over ten times lower than in the Cook Island population. Presumably, the Fijian diet is richer in gamma tocopherol than the Cook Islanders' diet, which may be reflected in the significantly lower incidence of lung cancer among the Fijians.

Several studies of smokers have found that cigarette smoking also depletes gamma tocopherol, and the gamma tocopherol levels in ex-smokers rise days after they cease smoking.

Similarly, a Swedish study found that gamma but not alpha tocopherol levels in serum were reduced in coronary heart disease patients. This discovery is particularly interesting in light of information recently proposed by California researchers that a natural diuretic produced by the body, LLU-alpha, is a metabolite of gamma tocopherol. Natural diuretics maintain the body's normal mineral balance and by doing so help protect it against high blood pressure. That means if you do not get enough gamma tocopherol, your body cannot produce enough of this natural diuretic. This could potentially be very serious, since high blood pressure increases the risk of both heart attack and stroke.

Smokers are also at higher risk of heart disease and stroke, and although it has never been studied, gamma tocopherol may help shield them from these diseases as well. Based on the studies that I cited earlier, gamma tocopherol appears to protect against lung cancer in smokers. How? Tobacco smoke contains large amounts of nitrogen dioxide, a compound that can be converted into a potential carcinogen. However, natural gamma tocopherol interacts with nitrogen dioxide and sends it down a different pathway, thereby preventing the formation of this carcinogen. At this point, this is largely speculation, but we may soon have concrete evidence of gamma tocopherol's protective power.

The Packer Lab is involved in a large intervention trial that will administer a network antioxidant cocktail rich in gamma tocopherols and tocotrienols to smokers in cooperation with the State of California Tobacco Research Disease Related Program. (The study is described in further detail on page 51.) In our study, the majority of vitamin E is delivered in the gamma form, but we will still include alpha tocopherol. This is in keeping with my belief that the best benefits of vitamin supplementation come when the supplement contains all the natural forms of vitamin E, not one to the exclusion of the other. It will be several years before we have the final results, but based on preliminary research, I am optimistic about the outcome. I don't mean to imply that we can protect smokers from all the risks associated with tobacco use, but I do believe we can reduce those risks through antioxidant supplementation.

As we learn more about gamma tocopherol, undoubtedly its health benefits will become more apparent, and there will be a growing recognition of the importance of the entire vitamin E family.

Vitamin E enhances immune function

It is not enough to extend life if those extra years are going to be wasted on illness; we must also find a way to preserve health. One way to preserve health—and to add life to our years—is to maintain a strong, vigorous immune system. In this regard, bolstering the antioxidant network can make a difference in our ability to ward off diseases that not only shorten life, but also disrupt our quality of life during those later years.

The primary job of the immune system is to protect our bodies against disease. Although we call it a system, the immune system is not associated with one particular organ. In reality, it is a collection of cells that seek out and destroy bacteria, viruses, precancerous and cancer cells, and any other foreign invader that it deems to be dangerous.

As we age, the immune system loses some of its punch, and as a result, we become more vulnerable to diseases that we could easily have shaken off in our youth. This is the reason why older people are strongly advised to get flu shots each year, and most younger people are not. Whereas a younger person could defeat the influenza virus in a week or two, an older person may not be as lucky. He is more likely to stay sick for a longer time and to have a greater risk of developing complications such as pneumonia.

There are several different types of immune cells. T-cells are the main cells of the immune system. Some T-cells circulate throughout the bloodstream, hunting down foreign invaders and protecting cells against direct attack from viruses and bacteria. Other T-cells, called suppressor cells, help immune cells distinguish between the cells of the body and foreign proteins. Suppressor cells are very important because if we didn't have them, the body could attack itself, causing serious damage to body organs and even death. A malfunction in suppressor cells can lead to autoimmune diseases such as systemic lupus erythematosus, Sjögren's syndrome, or rheumatoid arthritis.

Another type of immune cell, B-cells, produce proteins called antibodies that attach onto a foreign substance when it is introduced into the body. Throughout our lives, our bodies make thousands of different antibodies, each tailored to search out and destroy a particular enemy. Antibodies can hold a grudge for a long, long time. After defeating a foe, they remain in our bodies to vanquish viruses or bacteria should they dare to strike again. For example, most people will only get chicken pox once, because if the chicken pox virus tries to strike a second time, an army of antibodies will recognize it and attack it before it can take hold.

As we age, there is a measurable drop in immune function, especially by our seventh and eighth decades. Although we may produce as many T-cells and B-cells as we did before, they do not work as well. In fact, by the time we're seventy, no more than half of our T-cells are capable of responding to an antigen or foreign body. Our B-cells also begin to lose their memory and are no longer as aggressive in pouncing on our enemies.

In older animals and human cells, vitamin E can boost immune function, but until recently, there have not been any convincing studies showing a positive immune response in older people as a result of taking vitamin E. I am happy to report that researchers at Jean Mayer, USDA Human Nutrition Center at Tufts University, under the direction of Simin Nibkin Meydani, have proven that vitamin E not only works in test tubes and on laboratory animals but can stimulate immune function in older people as well.

In their study, eighty-eight people ages sixty-five plus were given either 60, 200, or 800 I.U. of vitamin E daily for four months. At the end of the four-month period, researchers reported the following:

* A significant increase in T- and B-cell activity in those who took vitamin E, a clear indication that they were better able to keep illness at bay than those who took a placebo.

* Those people who took vitamin E showed a more vigorous immune response to delayed hypersensitivity skin response, hepatitis B, and the tetanus vaccine.

* Study participants were also asked to keep track of all infections (such as colds, viruses, and sore throats) that occurred during the four-month period they were taking vitamin E. The people who took vitamin E reported a 30 percent lower incidence of self-reported infections than the people who did not take vitamin E.

Vitamin E: hope for Alzheimer's patients

Of all the diseases associated with aging, I believe that the one people fear the most is Alzheimer's disease, an irreversible form of dementia that is characterized by the slow, steady destruction of key areas in the brain. Typical symptoms include loss of memory and the inability to speak and process information. As the disease progresses, its victims lose awareness of themselves and others and often require round-the-clock care.

Some 4 million Americans have Alzheimer's disease, and experts predict that by 2020, that number could rise to over 10 million. Alzheimer's is a late-onset disease in that most of its victims are over sixty-five. In fact, about 10 percent of all Americans over age sixty-five have been diagnosed with Alzheimer's. However, in rare cases, it can strike people in their forties and fifties. There is no cure for Alzheimer's disease, although there are some drugs that may forestall the progress of the disease for some people.

Although we don't know the cause of Alzheimer's, we do know that it results in profound injury to brain tissue, notably the death of neurons, the worker cells of the brain. In particular, Alzheimer's is marked by the accumulation of a protein in the brain called *beta amyloid*. Since neural membranes are highly susceptible to oxidative damage, free radicals are also believed to be involved in the progression, if not the onset, of Alzheimer's disease as well as other degenerative brain diseases. The brain tissue of Alzheimer's patients typically has higher levels of lipid peroxidation, a sign of oxidative damage, than disease-free people of the same age. Many researchers suspect that free radical damage to neurons may inhibit the ability of nerve cells to produce adequate levels of neurotransmitters and other chemicals in the brain that organize thought processes and help brain cells communicate. As we get older, there is a natural decline in the production of neurotransmitters, which is a factor in normal brain aging. However, this decline may be greatly accelerated in the brains of Alzheimer's patients.

Animal and test tube studies have strongly suggested that vitamin E may play a role in preventing Alzheimer's disease by protecting brain cells against free radical attack. We have performed numerous experiments in my laboratory that demonstrate that vitamin E (along with Coenzyme Q10, the other fat-soluble antioxidant) can reduce lipid peroxidation in the brain. What's even more exciting is that a recent multi-institution double-blind, placebo-controlled study conducted by the Alzheimer's Disease Cooperative Study showed that vitamin E worked even better than standard drug therapy in treating Alzheimer's patients.

In this study, a total of 341 patients with early Alzheimer's disease of moderate severity were divided into four groups. The first group received 10 milligrams of selegiline, a monoamine oxidase inhibitor, daily; the second group was given 2000 I.U. of vitamin E daily; the third group was given both selegiline and vitamin E daily and the fourth group was given a placebo. The purpose of the study was to determine whether any of these therapies could slow down the progress of the disease so that patients would not deteriorate as rapidly. After two years, the researchers reported that the risk of reaching the most severe stage of Alzheimer's disease was 53 percent lower in the group taking vitamin E alone, 43 percent lower in the drug group, and 31 percent lower in the combination group than in the group taking the placebo. Of all these treatments, vitamin E alone worked the best.

Based on the growing number of studies that show vitamin E and other antioxidants can protect against so-called brain aging, vitamin E may prove to be useful in delaying the onset of Alzheimer's disease, or in some cases, even preventing it from occurring in the first place by protecting brain tissue against oxidative damage.

Exercise and antioxidants

If oxygen is a dangerous friend because it promotes the formation of free radicals, any activity that turns up the metabolic rate, that is, that causes you to burn more oxygen, could also put you at risk. Exercise is widely believed to be beneficial—and is—but it also has a potential downside.

First, the good news. Nearly all of us will benefit greatly from regular exercise, both physically and mentally. Exercise improves the cardiovascular system and the microcirculation, promotes a feeling of well-being, and in general, makes most people more aware of their diet and lifestyle. Regular exercise will undoubtedly contribute to healthier aging.

However, during exercise, oxygen consumption may rise several times as high as normal, and wherever oxygen is burned, there are free radicals. More than twenty-five years ago, two researchers in my laboratory, Kelvin J. A. Davies and Alexandre Quintanilha, were the first to show that free radicals are generated by physical exertion, and that vitamin E can protect against some of the damage produced by physical exercise.

In several experiments, we showed that after vigorous exercise on a treadmill, endurance-trained animals experienced an increase in free radicals and lipid peroxidation, and a decrease in glutathione, the classic scenario for oxidative stress. In particular, the animals had lower levels of vitamin E and telltale signs of injury to muscle cell membranes, another indication of free radical attack. However, when given vitamin E, the animals experienced far less oxidative stress and were actually able to exercise longer.

It's not just laboratory animals that need to worry about the potentially harmful effects of exercise. In Berkeley, we have performed several human studies (together with exercise physiologist George A. Brooks) that measured the effect of vigorous exercise, such as downhill running on a treadmill, on antioxidant levels. These studies have all confirmed that after a strenuous workout, there is an enormous decrease in blood glutathione levels and signs of lipid peroxidation, which means the body is in oxidative stress, and lipids and proteins are being damaged. After a period of exercise, the body repairs the damaged lipids and proteins, and about 99.9 percent are returned to normal. However, a tiny fraction will remain damaged, and over time, the accumulated damage can cause problems. That is why it is especially important for people who exercise regularly to have their antioxidant defenses in place to minimize the potential for damage.

Depending on the sport, vitamin E supplementation might not only protect against oxidative stress but may actually improve stamina and performance. In one study of high-altitude mountain climbers, those who regularly took 400 I.U. vitamin E supplements not only had better endurance but had less evidence of lipid peroxidation. When speed swimmers were supplemented with vitamin E, however, there was no effect on endurance. It is not fully understood why vitamin E may provide an energy boost for one group of athletes but not another. The bottom line is, even if vitamin E is not a "magic bullet" to enhance athletic performance for every sport, it offers significant long-term benefits in protecting against free radical damage.

Since so many people are embarking on exercise programs today to maintain their youth and vitality, I feel that these findings have not received the attention they should. I worry that in the long run, people who exercise who do not adequately bolster their antioxidant defenses may be doing themselves unnecessary harm. In particular, endurance athletes who place unusual demands on their bodies should be especially vigilant about maintaining their antioxidant advantage. Some coaches are poorly trained in exercise science, and there needs to be a better merger between exercise science and coaches and athletes to optimize physical exercise and the ability to exhibit superior performance. There also needs to be a greater concern about the long-term effect of exercise on the bodies of athletes, who may not be as careful about eating an antioxidant-rich diet or taking their supplements as they should be.

Parents of teenage athletes also need to understand the long-term effects of oxidative stress on their children, and to make sure that their teenagers begin taking vitamin E early in life to prevent problems down the road.

Vitamin E helps save your vision

Two-thirds of all Americans will have a cataract by age eighty-five. It need not happen. There is growing evidence that vitamin E may help to prevent this most common age-related vision problem. A cataract is a cloudy or opaque covering that grows over the lens of the eye, which can cause total or partial blindness. A cataract can distort vision by making objects look vague and fuzzy. If the cloudiness on the eye lens becomes so severe it hampers vision, the cataract must be surgically removed. Four million U.S. men and women have cataracts, and most people who have them are over the age of sixty. Cataracts are so commonplace in the United States that more than 10 percent of the Medicare budget is spent on cataract surgery. In rare cases, a cataract may be caused by a genetic problem, but the overwhelming majority of cases are caused by cellular damage to the eye lens inflicted by exposure to ultraviolet and visible light. The lens of the eye is particularly susceptible to light-induced lipid and protein oxidation, a major factor in the majority of cases of cataracts. The lens contains proteins called crystallins, which, when damaged, can become irregular and refract light in the wrong way, thereby leading to cataract formation.

There are several reasons why I am optimistic that vitamin E may prove to be a useful tool in the prevention of cataracts. First, numerous animal studies have shown that vitamin E can arrest and reverse the development of cataracts and can protect the sensitive lens tissue from oxidative damage. Second, population studies have documented that people with low blood levels of antioxidants E, C, and carotenoids are more likely to develop cataracts than those with higher levels. The third, and perhaps the most persuasive, bit of evidence is a recent study that actually contrasted the self-reported consumption of supplements by 175 cataract-free patients over age fifty-five to that of 175 patients of the same age group with cataracts. The cataract-free group used significantly more vitamins C and E than the group that already had developed cataracts. I think it is fair to say that even if vitamin E does not do the job alone, in combination with other network antioxidants it may offer powerful protection against cataracts.

Vitamin E helps heal arthritis and inflammation

Fifty million Americans suffer from some form of arthritis, an umbrella term for more than 100 different diseases that produce either inflammation of the connective tissue or the degeneration of articular cartilage. As the cartilage between the joints gets worn down, the bones become exposed, resulting in pain, stiffness, and swelling in the joints.

Although we don't know the cause of arthritis, long-term exposure to free radicals is believed to be a factor in either the initiation or progression of this potentially painful and debilitating disease. Several studies have shown that vitamin E can help reduce the symptoms of arthritis, and patients report a lessening of stiffness, improved mobility, and a decrease in the need for painkillers. Vitamin E not only helps to defeat free radicals but can also inhibit the biological pathway that triggers inflammation.

E is for everyone

There is an impressive body of work to support the role of vitamin E in maintaining optimal health. Today, virtually every scientific researcher in the field of aging and I would guess a good many physicians take vitamin E daily, even if they won't admit to it.

I firmly believe that taking vitamin E will not only extend life but will also enhance life. It is an essential component of the antioxidant network, and I wholeheartedly recommend it for everyone.

6

Vitamin C
The Hub of the Network

* People who take vitamin C supplements daily significantly reduce their risk of dying of cancer and heart disease.

* Vitamin C prevents cancer by shielding DNA from free radical damage.

* Vitamin C protects sperm from free radical damage. Men who are conceiving children should be vigilant about taking extra vitamin C daily.

* Vitamin C regenerates vitamin E and interacts with flavonoid antioxidants in the network.

* Touted as the cure for the common cold, vitamin C is critical for a well-functioning immune system. By strengthening immune function, vitamin C may reduce the length and severity of colds and viruses and bolster the body's ability to resist cancer.

* C is the vitamin for great skin. It is essential for the production of collagen, the cellular glue that holds the body together and keeps skin young and supple.

* Vitamin C works with E to prevent the oxidation of lipoproteins that can lead to heart disease.

* C protects against cataracts, a leading cause of vision problems among older people.

* *RDA:* 60 milligrams; 100 milligrams for smokers.

* *The Packer Plan:* 500 milligrams daily of ester C (250 milligrams A.M. and 250 milligrams P.M.).

* *Sources:* Vitamin C is abundant in plants and is present in many fruits and vegetables including red peppers, broccoli, cranberries, cabbage, potatoes, tomatoes, and citrus fruit.

I call vitamin C the hub of the antioxidant network because it is the link connecting the fat-soluble antioxidants to the water-soluble ones. In the network, vitamin C has the important job of recharging fat-soluble vitamin E when it becomes a free radical. Although lipoic acid can also regenerate E, vitamin C does it better.

Vitamin C is remarkably similar in molecular weight and structure to glucose, a simple sugar in the bloodstream that is used to make fuel to run the body. This gives vitamin C a decided advantage over the other network antioxidants. Energy is so essential to the functioning of the body that glucose is rapidly taken up by the cells. In other words, it is favored over other molecules trying to get into the cells. As you may remember, when a network antioxidant defuses a free radical, it then becomes oxidized into a weak free radical and must be recycled back to its antioxidant form. Since the oxidized form of vitamin C is almost identical to glucose, it gets a free ride on the glucose express and is also rapidly taken into the cells. Within the cells, oxidized C is recycled into antioxidant vitamin C and is returned to the plasma to protect proteins and lipoproteins.

Surprisingly, human beings are one of the few animals that do not produce vitamin C on their own and therefore must rely on getting enough of it through food or supplements. In this respect, we are similar to guinea pigs, the fruit-eating bat of India, and a songbird called the red vented bulbul, which all lack the necessary enzyme to convert glucose into vitamin C. By comparison, all other animals—from the common housefly to the family dog—produce relatively large amounts of vitamin C. For example, a goat produces as much as 13,000 milligrams of vitamin C daily, and some larger animals produce up to 20,000 milligrams of vitamin C daily.

Since humans and animals live in the same environment, breathe the same air, and are exposed to the same level of free radical attack, why we do not manufacture vitamin C has been the source of much speculation and debate. Some scientists theorize that the loss of the necessary enzyme was actually a genetic mistake that occurred around 45 million years ago. They argue that early primates were able to survive without making vitamin C because their diet was primarily vegetarian, and our ancestors consumed very high levels of vitamin C through fruits and vegetables. If our vegetarian ancestors subsisted on 2,500 calories daily in plant food, which is a rich source of vitamin C, it is possible that they were eating about 10,000 milligrams of vitamin C. In addition, freshly grown fruits and vegetables have a much higher vitamin C content than those that may travel thousands of miles before we actually eat them.

Today, most of us do not consume anywhere near the amount of vitamin C that our ancestors did. In fact, about 25 percent of the U.S. population does not consume the paltry 60 milligrams RDA for vitamin C every day. Smoking decreases the amount of vitamin C in the lungs and blood plasma, an indication that smokers are under additional oxidative stress that requires additional antioxidant support.

The scurvy saga

Throughout history, we humans have paid a steep price for our inability to produce vitamin C. If we do not get enough of this essential vitamin, we will succumb to scurvy, a deficiency disease characterized by bleeding gums, skin hemorrhages, severely weakened bones, and eventually death.

Long before we knew that vitamin C deficiency was the cause, scurvy was a particularly common occurrence on long sea voyages, where for months at a time, sailors would be forced to subsist on inadequate diets devoid of fresh fruits and vegetables. An occasional day without enough vitamin C is not going to cause scurvy, but three or four months without any vitamin C, as was common for sailors, was a veritable prescription for scurvy. It is estimated that more than a million seamen died from this disease during the seventeenth and eighteenth centuries alone. Explorers such as Vasco da Gama and Magellan reported losing more than half their crew to the painful and deadly disease.

Interestingly, it was once believed that scurvy was caused by physical exercise. The sailors who developed scurvy were typically those members of the crew who were sent ashore, while the ship's officers did not get sick. While on land, crew members often engaged in vigorous activity, such as pulling sleds laden with skins and pelts over miles of rough terrain back to the ship. Today we know that physical exertion produces free radicals, which in the case of these sailors quickly depleted whatever vitamin C they had left in their bodies.

As far back as 1227, an explorer named Gilbertus de Aguilla advised sailors to "carry an ample supply of apples, pears, lemons, and muscutals as well as other fruits and vegetables," to avoid this dreadful disease. Unfortunately, his advice was not heeded, because cases of scurvy continued to soar. The cure for scurvy was not officially recognized until the middle of the eighteenth century. In what is believed to be the first controlled study in any area of clinical science, British physician James Lind tested various popular treatments for scurvy. He selected twelve sailors with scurvy and divided them into six pairs, feeding each pair a different diet. Lind tried a number of different popular remedies, including extract of ginger, sulfuric acid, and vinegar solutions. Only the sailors he placed on two oranges and one lemon a day showed great improvement. In fact, within six days, they were ready to return to active duty. Lind was convinced that he had found the cure for the disease and possibly a way to prevent it, and reported his results in his book *A Treatise of the Scurvy*, published in 1753. It wasn't until he died, however, in 1795 that the British Admiralty finally adopted the use of citrus fruits—notably lemons and limes—in the prevention of scurvy (hence the nickname "limeys" for British sailors). In fact, it was a punishable offense for any sailor in the British navy to refuse his citrus ration.

Many researchers question why it took the British medical establishment four decades to accept Dr. Lind's findings. There are probably two reasons for this: First, it seemed improbable that such a deadly disease could be cured so quickly and simply through diet alone. This is not surprising—even today, physicians are reluctant to recognize the power of nutrition. Second, it can take several decades for an innovative idea to catch on, even if it's correct. History is replete with examples of innovative scientists being scorned in their own time. Louis Pasteur was considered insane by his colleagues for suggesting that disease was caused by invisible microorganisms. A more recent example of the resistance of the medical community to accept new concepts is the experience of two Australian researchers Dr. Barry Marshall and Dr. Robin Warren, who discovered that a bacterium called *H. pylori* causes most ulcers, and that most ulcers could be cured by treating them with antibiotics, not antacids. Although they had ample evidence to back up their claims, they were greeted by skepticism and ridicule by the medical community. Today antibiotics are the principal treatment for ulcers. So it is understandable that when physicians were told that oranges and lemons could cure the scourge of the seas, they, too, were skeptical.

Scurvy is very rare today, but it reappears during times of war and famine when fresh vegetables and fruits are scarce. For example, in the United States, scurvy reemerged in the large cities during the Great Depression and afflicted Allied troops during World War II. Recently, cases were reported in Somalia during their civil war in the 1980s.

The link between vitamin C and scurvy was not made until the twentieth century with the discovery of vitamin C. Although several other scientists laid the groundwork, Hungarian-born scientist Dr. Albert Szent-Györgyi (who recognized the importance of flavonoids) is first credited with isolating vitamin C from red pepper. For his efforts, he won the Nobel Prize in 1937. He called this new substance ascorbic acid (for "antiscorbutic") or vitamin C. Interestingly, the American Medical Association objected to the ascorbic acid name on the grounds that it sounded too much like a therapeutic drug; they proposed the name cetavitamic acid, but the name never caught on.

How much C is enough?

After the discovery of vitamin C, some researchers speculated that low levels of vitamin C may increase the risk of common infections and some physicians reported success in treating patients with high doses of vitamin C. Much of this work was stopped after the discovery of antibiotics in the 1940s, the wonder drugs that were supposed to wipe disease off the face of the earth.

More than seventy years later, vitamin C continues to be a cause of much controversy, mostly centering on one question: How much is enough? The modern debate began in the 1970s with the publication of *The Healing Factor: Vitamin C Against Disease* by biochemist Irwin Stone. Dr. Stone argued that because humans do not produce vitamin C, we are living in a state of vitamin C deprivation that makes us especially vulnerable to a plethora of diseases, including heart disease and cancer. Dr. Stone was the first scientist to suggest that people should ignore the low RDA for vitamin C, which is based solely on the amount needed to prevent scurvy, and recommended much higher doses—up to 200 times the RDA in some cases—to compensate for this deficiency.

The man who really put vitamin C on the map, however, was the late Dr. Linus Pauling, the two-time Nobel Prize winner (his first award was for chemistry, his second for peace) whose book *Vitamin C and the Common Cold* changed the way much of the public thought about vitamins. In his book, which was based largely on anecdotal reports and personal observation, Dr. Pauling reported that by taking 1 gram of vitamin C daily, it was possible to prevent the common cold. In addition, he promised that high doses of vitamin C would make you feel more alert and energized. If you already had a cold, Dr. Pauling recommended taking several grams of vitamin C a day until it was cured.

Vitamin C and the Common Cold generated great excitement for several reasons. First and foremost, colds are caused by viruses, and even though antibiotics such as penicillin and its offspring could conquer many bacterial infections, we still did not know how to combat a viral infection. If a simple vitamin could cure a cold, people hoped that it could also cure troublesome viruses such as the flu. Second, the public was growing disenchanted with conventional medicine that neglected such important factors as nutrition and lifestyle and totally ignored (and often disdained) what we now call preventive medicine. Right or wrong (or as I often say, Dr. Pauling was right, but for the wrong reasons) the world was ready for Dr. Pauling's message.

Dr. Pauling and his followers created a new field—orthomolecular medicine—which was based on the premise that nutrients and vitamins should not be used merely as a tool to prevent deficiency diseases but should be taken at the right doses necessary to achieve optimal health and even treat diseases. It was named after the Greek word *orthos,* which means correct.

Dr. Pauling's thesis elicited a strong response by much of the medical community that contended (without much evidence) that megadoses of C were dangerous and would result in an epidemic of serious health problems including kidney stones, vitamin B deficiency, and even "rebound scurvy," which might occur if people suddenly stopped taking high doses of vitamin C. The naysayers turned out to be wrong. Their admonitions did not stop millions of people from taking megadoses of vitamin C, with few ill effects. Because vitamin C is a water-soluble vitamin, any excess that is ingested is eliminated in urine. There is no chance for toxic buildup. The only negative effects from too much vitamin C are abdominal cramping and diarrhea, which are uncomfortable but not particularly hazardous to your health. In very rare cases, people with a defect in iron or folic metabolism may experience an adverse reaction to megadoses of vitamin C, but there have been few reported cases. As I see it, the real question is not whether megadoses of C have done any harm, but rather have they done any good?

It all depends on how much you take. First, I would like to state unequivocally that I believe that the RDA for vitamin C is much too low and does not provide adequate antioxidant protection. Here is some compelling evidence why:

* My colleagues, Bruce Ames and Billy Fraga, recently performed a study in which they showed that levels of vitamin C under 200 milligrams a day were not enough to protect DNA in sperm from oxidative damage. Human semen has eight times the vitamin C as present in blood, a clear indication that it plays an important role in preserving genetic integrity. Although the 60 milligrams RDA is adequate to prevent scurvy, it is not enough to prevent defective genes from being passed on to offspring.

* James E. Enstrom of the University of California studied 12,000 people over a ten-year period. In his study, the participants were asked to fill in a dietary questionnaire to evaluate vitamin C status. He divided the participants into three groups: those who consumed 0–50 milligrams of vitamin C daily, those who consumed more than 50 milligrams daily from food, and those who took regular vitamin C supplements in excess of 50 milligrams. After tracking these three groups for ten years, Dr. Enstrom found that those who fared the best in terms of staying disease-free and healthy were those who took more than 50 milligrams of C daily. What was truly remarkable, however, was the dramatically lower risk of death from heart disease, cancer, and mortality in

general from those who supplemented with C daily, typically taking well above the RDA.

✳ My colleague, Gladys Block, considered one of the leading experts in the world on vitamin C, has reviewed hundreds of studies examining the role of vitamin C or vitamin C–rich foods in the prevention of cancer, and the overwhelming majority found a direct relationship between an increased consumption of fruits and vegetables high in vitamin C and a lower incidence of cancer. The link was particularly strong for cancers of the esophagus, mouth, stomach, and pancreas.

Vitamin C and the cancer connection

It makes sense that vitamin C offers protection against oral and gastrointestinal cancers (as well as some others). Vitamin C protects against nitrosamines, cancer-causing agents found in food that may be responsible for initiating cancers of the mouth, stomach, and colon.

In recent years, vitamin C has been touted as a potential treatment for cancer. Much of these claims are based on Dr. Pauling's book, *Cancer and Vitamin C,* which is based on the experiences of Ewan Cameron, a Scottish physician, and Pauling in treating advanced cancer patients with very high doses of vitamin C, often in conjunction with other therapies. In most cases, the patients were in such an advanced state there was little else to do for them. In no case did either Dr. Cameron or Dr. Pauling suggest that a patient turn down a conventional treatment with a proven track record. In several cases, patients fared significantly better than expected when given vitamin C therapy. As interesting as the book may be, once again it is based largely on anecdotal evidence and not on the kind of clinical evidence mandated by science. Although we know that antioxidants may offer strong protection against many different forms of cancer, there is no firm evidence to date that they are of any benefit once you have the disease. Perhaps one day there will be, but until then, I would certainly not recommend that anyone reject conventional treatment in favor of antioxidant therapy if it is available.

Despite the controversy he generated, Dr. Pauling, who died at age ninety-three in 1994, not only had a profound effect on changing the public's perception of health care, but on the practice of medicine itself, which through the years has become more nutritionally oriented. When physicians today refer to themselves as practitioners of "integrative" or "holistic" medicine, and when they combine nutrition and supplements with other sound therapies, they are proof of Dr. Pauling's legacy.

I am certainly a fan of vitamin C and have the utmost respect for Dr. Pauling. This does not mean, however, that I advocate taking huge doses of it. For one thing, at the time Dr. Pauling presented his innovative ideas, we were not aware of the antioxidant network or that antioxidants work best when they work together. We now know that many of the benefits Dr. Pauling attributed to vitamin C are actually a result of vitamin C's enhancing effect on vitamin E. Armed with this new knowledge, I believe that the goal of orthomolecular medicine should be to achieve the right balance among the network antioxidants so that the body can operate the way nature intended.

I had an opportunity to talk with Dr. Pauling in 1993 when he was the commencement speaker at the University of California at Berkeley. Already well into his nineties, Dr. Pauling was vigorous, alert, and still one of the most creative thinkers of his time. Before the graduation ceremony, as we donned our caps and gowns, I described the antioxidant network to Dr. Pauling and the recent studies performed in my laboratory that had shown a synergism among these antioxidants. Although Dr. Pauling was intrigued by the concept, he was not convinced. To Dr. Pauling, the story began and ended with vitamin C.

I like to think that if Dr. Pauling had lived long enough to read this book, I might have made a convert out of him!

In reality, when it comes to vitamin C, less may be more in terms of bioavailability and absorption. What people often forget is that simply swallowing a vitamin pill does not guarantee that it will be absorbed into the system and delivered to the appropriate cells and tissues. One way to determine how much of a particular vitamin is actually being utilized by the body is to administer a specific dose, and then measure how much of the vitamin is passing through the urine in unchanged form. According to a recent study designed to test bioavailability, if you take a 180-milligram supplement of vitamin C, half of it will be excreted in urine without being changed. However, if you take 2,000 milligrams of vitamin C, 90 percent will be excreted without being changed. In other words, if you take too much, the body will reach its saturation point and will not accept any more of the nutrient. Although you may not be harming yourself by taking megadoses of C, you are probably wasting your time and money. That is why I believe that lower doses may be more effective and recommend taking only 250 milligrams of vitamin C twice daily to maintain a constant level. This gives your body an opportunity to absorb the maximum amount of vitamin C possible.

People who are in poor health and therefore under a great deal of oxidative stress may require somewhat higher doses of vitamin C, but we don't know precisely how much. Proponents of megadoses of vitamin C point out that when animals are under physical or emotional stress, their production of vitamin C can increase two- or threefold. Some alternative physicians routinely prescribe several grams a day to patients suffering from conditions such as heart disease, arthritis, and even cancer and contend that it is helpful either alone or along with other therapies. In fact, Dr. Pauling wrote about his experiences treating cancer patients in his last book, *Cancer and Vitamin C*. To a great extent, however, we must rely on anecdotal or observational reports because well-run clinical studies are scarce.

This is not to say that vitamin C has not been well studied—there are thousands of studies performed on vitamin C each year that confirm its importance and unique role in health.

Vitamin C is for collagen

Vitamin C's function in the body goes well beyond its role as a network antioxidant. It is essential for the production of mature *collagen,* a protein that forms the connective tissue that supports the *dermis,* the outer layer of skin. Collagen is necessary for the formation of ligaments, bones, and blood vessels. It is literally the cellular glue that holds the body together. When collagen production is disturbed, as in the case of severe scurvy, the skin becomes so flaccid and weak that it practically falls off the body. Collagen is also critical for wound healing, and doctors often recommend taking vitamin C supplements after surgery.

Because collagen is an integral part of cartilage and bone, some physicians prescribe very high doses of vitamin C to people suffering from arthritis. Generally, people report an improvement in symptoms, although there is no evidence that vitamin C can actually regrow cartilage. As I have discussed earlier, other antioxidants have also been used with some success to treat arthritis, and here is another case where I believe the entire network may be more effective than any one antioxidant on its own.

Linus Pauling may have thought of vitamin C as the cure for the common cold, but today it is being touted by cosmetic companies as the cure for the common wrinkle. There are several new vitamin C creams and potions on the market that promise to erase fine lines, minimize wrinkles, and in a word, rejuvenate skin. Beyond the hype, there is some solid scientific basis for these claims.

As we age, we experience a decline in collagen production. The smooth, taut skin of youth is replaced with sagging, wrinkled skin that shows signs of skin aging. UV radiation from the sun, which generates the formation of free radicals, is also a major factor in skin aging. All of the network antioxidants can help protect skin from UV damage, as I will discuss in chapter 15, The Packer Plan: Antioxidants for Healthy, Beautiful Skin.

Until recently, it was believed that the slowdown in collagen production was simply another inevitable part of aging. Today, we know that maintaining the antioxidant advantage can help prevent and perhaps even reverse some of the signs of skin aging. Several studies suggest that the topical application of vitamin C skin creams and lotions can actually stimulate the production of collagen and make skin look younger and fresher. For example, in a study performed at Duke University Medical Center, researchers examined the effects of vitamin C on collagen synthesis in skin cells from either newborns (three to eight days old) or older adults (seventy-eight to ninety-three years old). In both cases, the researchers reported that the cells grew at a faster rate and were thicker when grown with vitamin C. They found that vitamin C actually enhanced the production of collagen synthesis. These studies were used as the basis to launch a new skin-care line of topical vitamin C products that have become quite popular.

I don't disagree that vitamin C can help maintain youthful, healthy skin, but I also believe that it could work even better by combining it with vitamin E and Pycnogenol, a flavonoid antioxidant booster.

Vitamin C: the cold fighter

Even though vitamin C is being prominently featured at the cosmetic counter, its primary claim to fame is that it is a disease-fighting antioxidant. After Dr. Pauling's assertion that vitamin C was the cure for the common cold, I believe that many people began to think of vitamin C as a new wonder drug that could wipe out viruses. At the first sign of a cold, people still take huge doses of C in the belief that the cold will vanish. In most cases, however, it doesn't. Several studies confirm that vitamin C cannot prevent or cure a cold but may lessen the duration and severity of the cold. Therefore, if you take vitamin C, you may shake off your cold symptoms faster.

Although vitamin C and its effect on cold symptoms have been well studied, we simply do not know for sure why it may speed up recovery from a cold and perhaps other infections as well. It has been suggested that, similar to antibiotics, vitamin C may have antiviral and antibacterial properties. I think that given what we now know about antioxidants, this explanation is too simplistic. I believe that unlike a drug that kills a specific microorganism, vitamin C's primary effect in battling infection is probably its role in the antioxidant network in general, and the immune system in particular. When vitamin C enters the body, it is literally gobbled up by immune cells. In fact, there are 20 to 100 times the concentration of vitamin C in immune cells as in the blood. As I have already discussed, immune cells produce high levels of free radicals, which are used to attack viruses, fungi, bacteria, and other unwanted intruders in the body. The overproduction of free radicals, however, can cause destruction of the immune cells and eventually weaken the system. The presence of vitamin C pools in these cells strongly suggests that it is there to protect against free radical attack.

C WORKS THROUGH E   In the antioxidant network, vitamin C recycles E, which is a proven immune-enhancing agent. In the chapter on vitamin E, I devoted a good deal of time to explaining E's role in stimulating immune function. By recycling E, vitamin C may indirectly be giving the immune system an added boost to fight infection.

C SUPPRESSES VIRAL GENES   Several studies have shown that vitamin C can suppress the replication of viruses such as the rhinovirus (the one that causes a stuffy nose during a cold) and other similar viruses in cell cultures. Studies have also documented a decrease in the incidence of bronchitis, tonsillitis, and other common throat and lung ailments in schoolchildren who were given vitamin C supplements as opposed to those who were not. These findings may appear to confirm that vitamin C is a virus killer, but in my opinion, that is simply failing to see the forest for the trees. There is a much bigger picture to see here, and once again, it is related to our new knowledge of the expanded role that antioxidants play in our bodies.

In order for viruses to be activated, they need to have their genes turned on. If their genes are not turned on, the virus will lie dormant. There have been several intriguing reports documenting that antioxidants may block the activation of viral genes, and I believe that this newly discovered role for antioxidants may in part explain the C phenomenon.

C STRENGTHENS CONNECTIVE TISSUE   By stimulating the growth of collagen, vitamin C may help prevent viral invasion by strengthening the connective tissue, thereby making our cells better able to ward off viral attack. In other words, vitamin C may help to build a protective barrier between viruses and cells so that viruses are not allowed to enter.

Vitamin C and your cardiovascular system

Until recently, researchers have focused on vitamin C's role in fighting infection and have overlooked a function of vitamin C that may be even more critical—its role in preserving the health of the cardiovascular system. It is surprising that this role has been so overshadowed by vitamin C's other jobs because it is so important.

By bolstering vitamin E, vitamin C also protects against the oxidation of lipoproteins, the first step in a long cascade of events that lead to hardening of the arteries. Fats travel through the bloodstream on lipoproteins, balls that consist of lipid molecules, protein, and some antioxidants, including vitamin E. Lipoproteins are highly vulnerable to free radical attack. If a free radical attacks a lipoprotein, vitamin E will defend it by reducing the free radical and, by doing so, will become a free radical itself. If E remains a free radical, it will be lost to the antioxidant system, and the lipoprotein it protects will be defenseless against the next free radical it encounters. Fortunately, vitamin C can rescue the vitamin E radical. Water-soluble vitamin C travels through the bloodstream; when it encounters a lipoprotein, it curls up close to it or to the cell membrane, recharging the vitamin E radical. In addition, vitamin C can also defuse any free radicals that it encounters, helping the body maintain its antioxidant advantage.

Taking vitamin C supplements can reduce the risk of heart disease. According to the study conducted at the School of Public Health at

UCLA under the direction of James Enstrom, men who took 300 milligrams of vitamin C daily had a 45 percent lower risk of heart disease than men who took less than 49 milligrams daily. It seems obvious that people who consume the lowest levels of vitamin C are not giving their bodies the tools they need to protect themselves against free radicals.

If you need more evidence that vitamin C is a heart-healthy vitamin, let me refer you to a fascinating study conducted at the University of Maryland School of Medicine that created quite a stir when it was published in the *Journal of the American Medical Association* in 1997. The purpose of the study was to assess the short-term effect of a single high-fat meal on the functioning of the inner layer of an artery, the *endothelium*. Impairment of endothelial function can disrupt normal blood flow and is an early sign of heart disease. In the study, twenty healthy volunteers were given either a high-fat meal (consisting of 50 grams of fat), a low-fat meal (0 fat) or a high-fat meal and pretreatment with oral administration of 1,000 milligrams of vitamin C and 800 I.U. of vitamin E. After the meal, the researchers measured blood flow through the artery using an ultrasound device. They found that blood flow was negatively affected for up to four hours following the high-fat meal without supplements, but these negative changes did not occur in the people who ate the low-fat meal or in those who took supplements. By the way, this doesn't give you carte blanche to eat all the fat you want as long as you pop a vitamin pill before each meal. This test showed the effect of supplements on one high-fat meal, and we don't know whether it would have the same effect over the long term. I suspect that the sensible combination of watching your fat intake and taking your antioxidant network supplements will prove to be a one-two punch against heart disease.

Diabetics need more C

One common medical condition that greatly increases the risk of developing heart disease is diabetes. Because glucose and ascorbic acid are taken up by the same pathway by the cell, there are important implications for diabetics. Under these conditions vitamin C will be competing with glucose to gain entry into the cells, and glucose will win. That will leave the cells deficient in vitamin C, making them even more vulnerable to oxidative stress, and ultimately to heart disease. Taking vitamin C supplements along with other antioxidants, as well as eating an antioxidant-rich, sensible diet will help to tip the odds in your favor.

Vitamin C and cataracts

Perhaps Dr. Pauling would have encountered less controversy if he had called his book *Vitamin C and the Common Cataract*. There is a growing body of evidence to support the claim that vitamin C may reduce the risk of developing cataracts, and even the most skeptical of clinicians must now concede that antioxidants play a role in protecting vision.

For more than a decade, the USDA Human Nutrition Research Center at Tufts University has been investigating whether antioxidant vitamins could reduce the risk of developing cataracts. Using participants from the Nurses Health Study, USDA researchers identified women between the ages of fifty-six and seventy-one. Some had been taking vitamin C supplements since the early 1980s; others had not. Researchers gave eye examinations to 165 of the supplement users and to 136 of the women who did not use supplements. Although none of the women had yet been diagnosed with cataracts, 188 showed early signs of the disease. The researchers found that the women who did not take vitamin C were much more vulnerable to developing cataracts than those who took supplements. In fact, 60 percent of the early cataracts appeared in women who did not take vitamin C supplements. Women who took vitamin C for at least ten years were only 23 percent as likely to develop cataracts as women who did not. Keep in mind that the average daily vitamin C intake from food of the women who didn't take vitamin C was about 130 milligrams, which is twice as high as the RDA, but evidently not high enough.

I believe that something as simple as taking a vitamin C supplement daily can make a huge difference in terms of protecting against heart disease, keeping immune function strong, preventing cataracts, and even slowing down skin aging. These are good enough reasons to take vitamin C even if it doesn't actually cure the common cold.

7

Coenzyme Q10
The Heart-Healthy Antioxidant

* **F**at-soluble Coenzyme Q10 regenerates vitamin E in the antioxidant network.

* For more than two decades, Co Q10 has been used successfully to treat and prevent heart disease in Japan and by innovative U.S. physicians.

* Co Q10 rejuvenates brain cells and may help to prevent Alzheimer's and Parkinson's disease.

* Co Q10 is currently being investigated as a treatment for advanced breast cancer.

* Co Q10 is used to treat gum disease.

* *RDA:* None.

* *The Packer Plan:* 30 milligrams daily as part of the basic plan. An additional 50 milligrams daily for people at high risk of heart disease or stroke.

* *Sources:* Synthesized by the body; also found in seafood and organ meats.

Two of the primary reasons that I am writing *The Antioxidant Miracle* is to change the public perception of antioxidants and to show how these powerful natural substances can be useful well beyond their role in controlling free radicals. Co Q10 is an example of an antioxidant that has been put to the test by innovative researchers and physicians and has passed with flying colors. This remarkable antioxidant is finally beginning to attract the attention it deserves, and although it is not yet as well-known as vitamins E and C, I predict that it will soon be an important part of a health-conscious lifestyle.

Before I tell you more about this exciting antioxidant, let me clarify a few facts. Co Q10 is a *coenzyme*. An *enzyme* is a protein found in living cells that brings about chemical changes; a coenzyme works *with* an enzyme to produce a particular reaction.

There are several molecular forms of Coenzyme Q in nature that vary according to the number of carbon atoms. At the base of the coenzyme is a *quinone*, a molecule that closely resembles vitamin E, to which is attached a long tail of carbon atoms in units of five. Coenzyme Q10 has ten units of carbon atoms, or fifty carbons; Coenzyme Q9 has nine units of carbon atoms, or forty-five carbons; Coenzyme Q8 has eight carbon units, or forty carbons, and so on. What's noteworthy about all of them is that the shortest-lived species (bacteria, insects, mice, and rats) have the shorter forms of Co Q, but only the longest-lived species—human beings and other large mammals—have Co Q10.

Co Q10 is involved in the Krebs cycle, the mechanism in which the body produces ATP or fuel. In fact, Co Q10 has been dubbed the "cellular spark plug" because just as a spark plug is needed to start the engine of an automobile, Co Q10 is essential for the production of energy that keeps the body running. Simply put, without enough Co Q10, you are running on empty.

Co Q10 is present in all cell membranes. It is so abundant within the cells that it is also known by the name *ubiquinone*, derived from the word *ubiquitous*. Co Q10 is found in highest amounts in the mitochondria, the energy-producing apparatus of virtually every cell, especially in the mitochondria of the heart, brain, kidneys, and liver, the hardest-working tissues of the body. It is there for a good reason.

In the mitochondria, Co Q10 serves two important functions. First, as I mentioned earlier, it is essential for making ATP. Second, Co Q10 is a fat-soluble antioxidant. At the same time cells are producing energy, they are also creating free radicals. In this capacity, Co Q10 serves double duty. It not only revs up energy production in the cells, but it can help quench troublesome free radicals.

But, even more important, Co Q10 recycles vitamin E, the most powerful fat-soluble antioxidant in the body. Work carried out in the Packer Lab by Valerian Kagen, Elena Serbinova, and John Maguire showed precisely how this is done and helped to highlight the importance of this once overlooked antioxidant. Along with vitamin E, Co Q10 is part of the antioxidant defense network that rides on the lipoprotein train throughout the bloodstream, protecting lipids from free radical attack.

In test tube studies, we have found that Co Q10 can regenerate vitamin E. We have duplicated these results in cultures of human skin, which suggests that along with vitamin E, Co Q10 offers protection against UV radiation, the leading cause of both skin aging and skin cancer.

Recently, Enrique Cadenas of the University of Southern California has discovered that nitric oxide, a free radical, reacts with Co Q10. Although the significance of this discovery is not fully understood, it suggests to me that Co Q10 could have an antioxidant action that has previously gone unrecognized.

Like many other substances produced by the body, levels of Co Q10 decline with age. Although Co Q10 is found in food such as salmon, liver, and other organ meats, it is nearly impossible to get enough Co Q10 from diet alone, especially in our later years. That is why I recommend that everyone over forty take 50 milligrams of Co Q10 daily. People with heart disease have lower Co Q10 levels than normal; therefore, I recommend an additional 50 milligrams daily as part of their supplement regimen.

Co Q10 was first discovered by Prof. Fred L. Crane at the University of Wisconsin in 1957, who isolated a mysterious orange substance from the mitochondria of beef hearts. Renowned physician and scientist Karl Folkers, who was the first to identify the structure of vitamins B_6 and B_{12}, isolated Co Q10 from beef hearts in 1958 when he was a research scientist at Merck, Sharpe and Dohme, the pharmaceutical giant. Although he immediately recognized the potential therapeutic importance of Co Q10, Dr. Folkers was unable to continue his research at Merck. For one thing, natural substances cannot be patented, so there is little financial incentive to pursue them. For another, the process of making Co Q10 from beef hearts was prohibitively expensive. Merck decided to sell the technology to produce Co Q10 to the Japanese, who later developed a more cost-effective method of producing natural Co Q10 by fermentation.

In 1965, a Japanese physician first used Co Q10 to treat congestive heart failure, a disease that is characterized by a heart that is too weak to pump blood properly. It worked. Today, some 6 million Japanese take Co Q10, where it is widely used as a treatment for heart disease and common ailments such as gum disease.

Fortunately, Dr. Folkers continued his research on Co Q10 at the University of Texas, where he made many more important break-throughs that have the potential to benefit the lives of many people. Dr. Folkers won virtually every chemistry award possible, and he even received the President's Medal of Science in 1990. He died at age ninety-one in December 1997, still actively involved in his work. Much of what we know about Co Q10 today, we owe to Dr. Folkers. These few words I wrote to Professor Gian Paolo Littarru, president of the newly formed Internal Coenzyme Q10 Association, upon hearing about Folkers's death best express my feelings toward this remarkable man. "Professor Karl Folkers was a true pioneer, a great scholar, scientist, and person. He will be badly missed from a research generation that is left behind with the fondest of memories." He will also be remembered by generations to come who will benefit from his work.

Dr. Folkers was the first to suggest that the age-related decline in Co Q10 was a contributing factor to many of the illnesses normally associated with aging, notably heart disease, cancer, and Alzheimer's disease. He reasoned that since energy is so important to the function of virtually every system in the body, it is impossible for any system to run well or efficiently if it is not getting adequate fuel. Since Co Q10 is involved in the production of ATP, it made sense that a decline in the production of this antioxidant would disrupt the body's energy-producing system. The effect of a shortage in energy would be felt by every system, from the cardiovascular to the immune to the repro-ductive.

Dr. Folkers laid the groundwork for numerous studies that showed that Co Q10 is a promising treatment for angina, congestive heart fail-ure, and cardiomyopathy. Before his death, Dr. Folkers also participated in two remarkable studies that reported some success in using Co Q10 as a treatment for advanced breast cancer.

To date, Co Q10's primary successes appear to be in the field of heart disease. Cutting-edge physicians have already begun to incorporate Co Q10 in their treatment regimens for heart disease. As you will see, there have been several important studies that have documented the benefits of Co Q10 for heart patients, which I will review here.

Your heart is one of the most hardworking organs in your body. Its job is critical—it pumps blood to the other vital tissues and organs. Your heart beats or contracts about 60 times a minute, 100,000 times a day, or 2.5 billion times during a normal life. Its beating is orchestrated by a superbly coordinated sequence of electrical impulses that begin within the heart itself. Your heart will beat whether you are sleeping or awake; in times of physical or emotional stress, you may make greater demands on your heart. Heart cells are so hardworking that if you remove them from the body and grow them in culture, they will continue to beat. Unlike most other muscles, the heart never gets to rest for prolonged periods.

The heart muscle contains 2 million heart cells, or *myocytes,* that are producing the energy required to run this active organ. The heart is a virtual hotbed of activity that requires a constant fuel supply.

When there is an inadequate supply of fuel, the heart will become sluggish. The primary cause of heart disease is atherosclerosis, a blockage in one of the arteries delivering blood to the heart. By blocking the flow of blood, it is depriving the heart of the nutrients it requires to produce enough energy to keep it pumping.

Heart patients often have dangerously low levels of Co Q10, an indication that they lack the "spark plug" required to keep the heart running normally. In fact, heart muscle biopsies in patients with various heart diseases showed a Co Q10 deficiency in 50 to 75 percent of all cases.

Since heart disease is often linked to deficiency in Co Q10, it seems reasonable to theorize that replenishing Co Q10 may have positive results. Several well-run studies performed in the United States and abroad suggest that it does for many patients. Most of this research was performed under the auspices of Karl Folkers at the Institute for Biomedical Research at the University of Texas, and cardiologist Peter Langsjoen of the Langsjoen Clinic, Tyler, Texas.

In one study conducted over an eight-year period (1985–1993) at the Langsjoen Clinic, 424 patients with cardiovascular disease were treated with Co Q10 along with their regular medication. These patients had a variety of ailments ranging from cardiomyopathy (injury to heart tissue) to high blood pressure to valve problems. Co Q10 doses varied from 75 to 600 milligrams daily. Patients were followed for nearly eighteen months. At the end of the study, researchers evaluated the patients' progress based on the New York Heart Association's (NYHA) rating for degree of illness, which is considered the gold standard throughout much of the world. The NYHA divides the stages of heart disease into four classes, class I being the least serious to class IV being the most serious. Out of the 424 patients, Dr. Langsjoen's group reported that more than half showed improvement by one NYHA standard, 28 percent by two classes, and 1.2 percent by three classes. What was truly remarkable was that during the study, nearly half of the patients stopped taking between one to three heart medications, a sign that they were improving. Unlike other heart medications that can cause a rash of unpleasant side effects, patients experienced virtually no side effects with Co Q10. The bottom line is that by including Co Q10 in the treatment of heart patients, there were a great many benefits, and no apparent negative side effects.

This is not the only study that has yielded positive results. In another study conducted by Dr. Langsjoen and Dr. Folkers, patients with cardiomyopathy, a serious condition that can lead to heart failure, were given Co Q10 along with other medication, Co Q10 alone, or medication without Co Q10. What was truly astonishing was that the patients taking Co Q10 with or without other drugs lived on average three years longer than those who were not taking Co Q10.

Japanese researchers have also found Co Q10 is a boon for heart patients, often speeding up their recovery. In one study conducted at the Hamamatsu University School of Medicine, ten men and two women with chronic unstable angina (chest pain) were recruited to participate in the twelve-week study, which was divided into three phases. In phase I, patients were given a placebo. In phase II, half of the patients were given a placebo and the others were given 50 milligrams of Co Q10 three times daily. In phase III, the group on the placebo was given Co Q10. During each phase, exercise tests on a treadmill were performed on each patient. Patients taking Co Q10 had reduced the frequency of anginal episodes by 53 percent, were able to exercise longer on the treadmill, and required less nitroglycerin for pain than those taking the placebo. Granted, this is a very small study, but given the result, it is certainly an indication that more studies are warranted.

In Italy, Co Q10 is routinely administered along with other cardiac drugs for congestive heart failure, and researchers report good results. In congestive heart failure, the heart does not pump efficiently and blood is not distributed properly throughout your body. Symptoms include extreme fatigue, swelling in the extremities, as well as heart palpitations, dizziness, and other unpleasant symptoms. In advanced cases, people with congestive heart failure are so exhausted that merely getting up from a chair can take great effort. In one Italian study involving 2,664 patients with congestive heart failure taking Co Q10 along with other medication, 54 percent showed an improvement in at least three symptoms of their disease, in addition to showing an improvement in the clinical signs of their disease, such as less edema or water retention and lower blood pressure, as well as in subjective symptoms. For example, 75 percent reported that they were less bothered by heart palpitations and sweating, 73 percent felt less tired, and 63 percent were able to sleep better at night. The patients taking Co Q10 said that they felt better. The researchers concluded that patients taking Co Q10 experienced an improvement in the quality of their lives.

There is one group of heart patients who absolutely should take Co Q10: those who are taking statin drugs such as lovastatin to lower their cholesterol. These drugs inhibit the synthesis of Co Q10 in the body, and this can be life-threatening for patients suffering from cardiomyopathy. Anyone taking these drugs should talk to their cardiologists about using Co Q10.

I am not suggesting that Co Q10 is a cure-all for heart disease. There is evidence, however, that along with other conventional therapies, it may speed up the recovery of heart patients, as well as make life more tolerable. My hope, of course, is by teaching people how to maintain the antioxidant advantage, we will be able to prevent many cases of heart disease from occurring in the first place.

Co Q10: a possible cancer aid

In 1971, President Richard Nixon declared war on cancer and stated that the country that eradicated polio and sent a man to the moon should easily be able to defeat this deadly disease. Almost three decades and billions of dollars later, we now know that cancer has proven to be a far more difficult adversary than originally believed. For one thing, cancer is not one disease, but an umbrella term for many different diseases, all characterized by the abnormal growth of cells. The cancer process begins when an errant cell mutates—i.e., it undergoes a change and begins to multiply wildly. These bad cells grow and invade neighboring groups of cells, robbing them of their nutrients. As cancer spreads, it invades various organ systems, making it impossible for the body to function normally.

Despite decades of research, there is still no magic bullet for cancer. In fact, the incidence of many different forms of cancer is on the rise. Today, one out of three North Americans will get cancer at some point in their lifetime, and beyond 2000, that number could rise. Although we have made significant strides in developing new therapies, we still can't answer the most fundamental question: What causes this disease? There are numerous theories, most of them involving free radical damage to genetic material within the cells, but few concrete answers. There is good evidence that a combination of genetics and environment is involved. For example, in women, a particular gene has been identified with an increased risk of breast cancer, and another gene has been implicated in an increased risk of prostate cancer in men. What is particularly confounding, however, is that many people get cancer who do not have these genetic markers, nor do all carriers of cancer genes go on to develop the disease. In fact, the National Cancer Institute estimates that at least half of all cases of cancer are caused by environmental factors such as smoking, diet, excessive alcohol intake, and lack of exercise. It is no coincidence that deaths from lung cancer among women have skyrocketed in the past decade, making it the number one cancer killer of women. After World War II, women began to smoke in unprecedented numbers. Each puff of smoke contains thousands of poisonous free radicals, which over time can destroy delicate lung tissue. We are just beginning to see the full impact of cigarette smoking in terms of female mortality, and as more and more young women take up smoking, I am afraid that this problem will plague us well into the twenty-first century.

I believe that antioxidants may prove to be effective in the prevention of cancer and may even be useful in the treatment of this disease along with other therapies. As we learn more about antioxidants, we are discovering the bigger role they play in keeping us healthy. We now know that not only do antioxidants keep free radicals under control, but even more important, they can also activate or suppress genes that control cell growth. It may soon be possible to harness the power of antioxidants in chemotherapy drugs designed to turn off the genes that trigger the growth of cancer. Of course, by maintaining the right level of antioxidants in your body, you may be protecting yourself against developing cancer in the first place.

When I discuss the role that antioxidants may play in cancer prevention, I don't want to suggest that simply popping a pill is the answer. There is overwhelming evidence, however, that eating a diet rich in fresh fruits and vegetables may offer powerful protection against cancer. Of course, fruits and vegetables are a major source of antioxidants and fiber as well as phytochemicals that we may not yet have discovered. My advice is, even if you take your supplements daily, be vigilant about eating a healthy diet.

Of all the different types of cancer, women most fear getting breast cancer. More than 200,000 American women are diagnosed with breast cancer each year, resulting in 46,000 deaths annually, making it the second leading cause of cancer deaths among women. If breast cancer is diagnosed early, the prognosis is excellent, but if it is diagnosed in its later stages, it is far more difficult to treat, and the outcome is less predictable.

Recently I learned of two Danish studies involving the use of Co Q10 on women with advanced breast cancer that offered a glimmer of hope to women with this problem.

In 1991, Karl Folkers reported that cancer patients had lower levels of Co Q10 in their blood than control subjects. Other studies had shown that Co Q10 boosted the effectiveness of T-cells, the body's disease-fighting immune cells that are involved in weeding out cancer cells. Dr. Folkers suggested that because cancer patients may not be able to produce Co Q10 efficiently, their body's ability to recover from the disease could be hampered.

In 1993, Dr. Folkers, along with researchers at a cancer treatment center in Denmark, ran a study on breast cancer patients. They selected thirty-two typical patients (ages thirty-two to eighty-one) designated high risk because their tumors had spread beyond the primary site to their lymph nodes. In addition to surgery and other conventional treatments, patients also received 90 milligrams of Co Q10 daily, along with a combination of other antioxidants, vitamins, minerals, and essential fatty acids. Before the study began, based on the serious condition of the women, researchers believed that there would be at least four deaths before the study was completed.

The results were remarkable. None of the women died; in fact, none of the patients showed signs of further distant metastases. All of the women reported no additional weight loss and a reduced use of painkillers. Six of the women showed signs of partial remission; in other words, their cancer was retreating. Since the women not only had conventional therapy but also took other antioxidants and vitamin supplements, the researchers noted that they could not attribute the positive result solely to Co Q10, but they noted that the combination of nutritional substances may have proven to be the key to achieving this successful outcome.

In a follow-up study, the Danish group selected three advanced breast cancer patients and prescribed 390 milligrams of Co Q10 daily. According to the physicians conducting the study, all of the women in this study fared surprisingly well.

Obviously, these are small studies, and the evidence is largely anecdotal. It would be imprudent to jump to any conclusions based on a handful of cases, and it would be equally foolhardy to eschew conventional treatment on the basis of these small studies. If a woman is interested in taking Co Q10 along with conventional therapy, she should only do so under the supervision of a physician, preferably one who routinely uses antioxidants in his or her practice.

I don't want to leave you with the impression that I believe that Co Q10 alone is responsible for the good results reported by the physicians who prescribe it to their patients. Since Co Q10 regenerates vitamin E, it is possible that the primary benefit of Co Q10 may be in its ability to boost the effectiveness of vitamin E. I suspect that an even more effective approach would be to use a combination of network antioxidants.

These preliminary studies highlight the need for good, carefully designed clinical trials to determine whether Co Q10 or any of the network antioxidants may be useful in either the treatment or prevention of breast cancer. Unfortunately, because Co Q10 and the other network antioxidants are not patentable, it is highly unlikely that a pharmaceutical company would be willing to fund such expensive studies. Until there is more scientific evidence, it is also unlikely that the National Institutes of Health would be willing to undertake this project.

A word of caution: Not all cancer patients should use antioxidants, at least while they are in the midst of treatment. Some chemotherapy drugs are designed to increase levels of disease-fighting free radicals to knock out cancer cells. Check with your physician before taking any supplements if you are undergoing chemotherapy.

Co Q10 rejuvenates the brain

In 1997, I was interviewed on the ABC *Nightly News* about cardiologist Peter Langsjoen's remarkable work with Co Q10. During that interview, I noted that if Co Q10 had a beneficial effect on the heart by enhancing the ability of the mitochondria to produce energy, I predicted that Co Q10 may prove to be important in "other disorders where defects in energy production occur, like Alzheimer's, Huntington's, and Parkinson's disease."

Simply put, the normal production of energy by brain cells is essential for normal brain function. Since Co Q10 is instrumental in the ability of mitochondria to produce energy, it should also help to slow down or even reverse some of the common age-related brain disorders.

Recently, I learned of a study that confirmed what I had predicted. Under the direction of Dr. Flint Beal, researchers at Massachusetts General Hospital gave laboratory mice a toxic drug called malonate, which kills brain cells by destroying mitochondria. These mice were also specially bred to develop amyotrophic lateral sclerosis (ALS), also known as Lou Gehrig's disease, a degenerative nerve disease that is characterized by an abnormally low level of antioxidants in the brain and an increase in free radical formation. In a sense, Dr. Beal had developed a model of accelerated brain aging, which is characterized by too few antioxidants, too many free radicals, and mitochondria that have grown sluggish.

When given a single injection into the brain containing the poison malonate, ALS mice will eventually develop big lesions in their brains that rapidly destroy brain tissue, leading to rapid death. However, when Dr. Beal administered Co Q10 along with the malonate, the mice showed substantially less brain damage and lived an average of eight days longer.

This proved that Co Q10 was able to provide protection for brain cells under the most trying conditions of oxidative stress. To me, this suggests that Co Q10 may also protect against other brain diseases associated with aging and the slowdown in mitochondrial function.

Co Q10 and healthy gums

I am willing to wager that most of you do not associate healthy teeth and gums with maintaining the antioxidant advantage, but what I am going to tell you may change your mind.

Call it the American paradox. Thanks in large part to fluoridated water and improved oral hygiene, Americans are getting fewer cavities. However, gum disease, which can lead to loss of teeth, is still very common in the United States. According to a 1985–1986 National Adult Dental Health Study, nearly half of all American adults had bleeding gums, a sign of inflammation, and 24 percent of all adults and 68 percent of all elderly people had significant periodontal attachments in their mouth (such as bridgework and caps), often caused by tooth loss. Gum disease is usually caused by the accumulation of bacterial plaque near the gum line, which causes gums to become inflamed. If the gum disease advances, it can destroy connective tissue and the bones supporting the teeth. In its end stages, there are frequently severe infections and tooth loss. Some 30 million Americans have gum disease, and nearly every adult over sixty-five has suffered some form of this problem. Antibiotics and other treatments, such as gum irrigation, are often used successfully to treat gum disease, but there is growing evidence that antioxidants may also be useful.

Gum disease usually strikes from midlife on because older tissue does not repair itself as quickly or efficiently as younger tissue. Some researchers speculate that the decline in the aging cell's ability to manufacture energy could be responsible for the body's inability to heal as rapidly. In addition, collagen that supports gum tissue is destroyed by free radicals, which has a cumulative effect. Since Co Q10 is involved in energy production and is an antioxidant, Japanese researchers have studied it as a possible treatment for gum disease.

As early as 1971, Japanese researchers discovered lower than normal levels of Co Q10 in the gum tissue of patients with gum disease and suggested that Co Q10 may be an effective treatment for gum disease. In fact, when Co Q10 was applied directly to the gums, and/or taken as a supplement, patients showed marked improvement and healed much more rapidly than those who did not use Co Q10. In an open trial conducted in the United States, patients undergoing periodontal surgery who took Co Q10 recovered up to three times faster than those who did not.

Co Q10 is a popular treatment for gum disease in Japan and is often included in toothpaste and mouthwash. Co Q10 gum-care products are now sold in the United States in health food stores.

Recently, studies have shown that the entire antioxidant defense network may be a factor in gum disease, not just Co Q10. In fact, researchers in Birmingham, England, found that patients with gum disease have lower levels of antioxidants in their saliva (but not blood serum) than patients without gum disease. Since inflammation is believed to be involved in the onset and progression of gum disease— and since free radicals are a by-product of inflammation—it makes sense that people who suffer from gum disease may not have as strong antioxidant defenses as those who don't. For example, smokers, who inhale thousands of free radicals with every puff, are at greater risk of developing serious gum disease. So are diabetics, who are also under a tremendous amount of oxidative stress. It makes sense that boosting the entire antioxidant network may help to prevent gum disease as well as other age-related ailments.

Whenever an antioxidant begins to attract media and public attention, as in the case of Co Q10, there is a tendency to focus solely on the one miracle cure. While it is true that Co Q10 has produced some encouraging results in the treatment of a wide variety of ailments, it is important to remember that it is not just Co Q10 at work, but the entire antioxidant network that is producing these miracles.

8

Glutathione
Nature's Master Antioxidant

* **K**eep your levels of glutathione high! Low levels of glutathione are a harbinger for illness and premature death.

* Produced in the body, glutathione is the primary water-soluble antioxidant. In the antioxidant network, glutathione recycles the oxidized form of vitamin C, restoring its antioxidant power.

* Lipoic acid can boost levels of glutathione.

* Glutathione is instrumental in the detoxification of drugs and pollutants and for healthy liver function.

* Glutathione is important for a strong immune system. Boosting glutathione can reverse age-related slump in immune function.

* Glutathione is involved in the storage and transport of amino acids, the building blocks of protein.

* *RDA:* None.

* *The Packer Plan:* The best way to boost glutathione levels is to take 100 milligrams of lipoic acid daily.

✸ *Sources:* Glutathione is abundant in fruits, vegetables, and freshly cooked meat, but it is broken down during digestion.

Although all of the network antioxidants are important, be especially vigilant about maintaining high levels of glutathione. Your life may depend on it.

Glutathione is present in the body in two forms: its reduced form, which is a potent antioxidant, and its oxidized form after it has been "used up" by the antioxidant defense network. In a healthy body, more than 90 percent of glutathione will be found in its antioxidant form. During times of illness or stress, however, levels of glutathione will plummet, a sign of oxidative stress.

In fact, low levels of glutathione are a marker for disease and death at any age. In patients with AIDS, people with the lowest levels of glutathione have the highest rate of mortality.

Why is glutathione so important? Glutathione is the cell's primary antioxidant. Found in the cell sap (the watery portion of the cell), there are several million times more glutathione molecules in the cells than vitamin E, the primary fat-soluble antioxidant. There are astonishingly high quantities of glutathione in the liver, where drugs, pollutants, alcohol, and other foreign substances are detoxified. Glutathione is so important that to be sure that we have enough of this precious antioxidant on hand, nature has devised a backup system within the body. Not only is glutathione constantly produced by cells, but it is also tucked away in proteins; this reservoir of extra glutathione will be mobilized into action under conditions of oxidative stress.

Similar to lipoic acid, glutathione is a thiol antioxidant, which means it contains a sulphur group. As you will see, there is a strong bond between these two sister antioxidants.

Glutathione is produced in the cells from three amino acids— cysteine, glutamic acid, and glycine—all of which can be derived from food. Glutathione is the only network antioxidant of which I do not recommend taking supplements. Although glutathione is sold as a supplement, there is much debate over how much glutathione actually passes through the intestine into the cells. Since glutathione is a large molecule, it was once believed that it was too large to pass intact from the digestive system into the cells. We now know that small amounts of glutathione may pass from the gastrointestinal tract to the bloodstream, but probably not in a high enough concentration to be helpful, and certainly not enough to be transported to the cells that need it.

Glutathione is so important that whenever your body is under oxidative stress, it immediately responds by producing a series of enzymes that are essential for glutathione production. Nevertheless, it is difficult for your body to keep up with the never-ending demand for glutathione, especially in times of illness.

So how can you ensure that you have enough of this lifesaving antioxidant? One of the most exciting discoveries made in the Packer Lab is that lipoic acid supplements can significantly boost levels of glutathione in target tissues where it is needed. In fact, I believe that some of the beneficial effects attributed to lipoic acid may be caused by its ability to increase glutathione. This would be in keeping with my overall philosophy that the network antioxidants are meant to work together, and it is often difficult, if not impossible, to tease out where one ends and the other begins.

There's a point of confusion here I'd like to clear up. You may have heard that taking the amino acid *N*-acetyl-L-cysteine (NAC), a precursor of cysteine, can increase glutathione levels. It does, but not nearly as well as lipoic acid. In fact, you have to take much higher doses of NAC to achieve the same result. In addition, NAC does not offer all the other benefits that can be achieved by taking lipoic acid. There are also analogs (synthetic versions) of glutathione that are available by prescription that if administered by injection have also been shown to increase glutathione levels. These drugs, however, are not generally available to the public. To my way of thinking, the easiest and best way to maintain optimal glutathione levels is to eat foods that contain the building blocks of glutathione, and to take a lipoic acid supplement.

It is also wise to avoid glutathione busters, the environmental toxins that can sap our glutathione. These include cigarette smoke and overly processed chemical-laden foods, such as luncheon meats that contain nitrites or nitrates. The excessive intake of alcohol will also deplete glutathione, which is one of the primary ways that too much alcohol can wreak havoc on the body. So can the common painkiller acetaminophen, as well as other over-the-counter and prescription drugs. You may remember that recently consumers were warned not to mix acetaminophen with alcohol. Both of these substances generate the production of free radicals. When combined, they can be pure poison to the liver by severely depleting the liver of glutathione. Without glutathione, the liver cannot function properly, which will result in a buildup of toxins that can cause liver poisoning.

I am writing about glutathione last not because it is the least important of the network antioxidants—far from it—but because it is the one that is hardest to study as a single antioxidant. Because it is so difficult to administer, there have not been as many "in vivo" studies in either animals or humans on glutathione as on the other network antioxidants. In fact, most of the studies on glutathione have been conducted either on cells in test tubes or on subjects who have been given drugs known to boost glutathione levels. In many cases, these drugs do not deliver glutathione efficiently to the tissues of the body. This makes it very difficult to study the effect of glutathione administration, which is why good studies on this antioxidant are difficult to obtain.

Glutathione was discovered well over a hundred years ago, but it has been only in the past few decades that scientists began to understand the crucial role it plays in health. Since high quantities of glutathione are found in the lens of the eye, the early research focused primarily on vision. Although glutathione may be critical for good vision, as are other antioxidants, we now know that it performs so many vital roles in the body that it has been dubbed "nature's master antioxidant" by my friend and colleague, the late Alton Meister, a well-known authority on glutathione.

Glutathione is certainly one of the network's busiest antioxidants. It performs many jobs far and above its role as traditional antioxidant. Here is a review of some of the things it does.

Glutathione gives your cells a fighting chance

Glutathione can help protect your cells against the kind of damage that can lead to cancer. One of glutathione's primary jobs is to rid the body of hydrogen peroxide, which is produced when fats and proteins become oxidized or damaged by free radicals. Hydrogen peroxide is not a free radical itself, but it can react with other substances such as iron to produce very reactive and potentially dangerous hydroxyl radicals. As you may recall, hydroxyl radicals are particularly nasty because they are practically unstoppable and can damage healthy cells and tissues. If cellular DNA is damaged and not repaired, it can cause the cell to mutate and lead to cancer. The best approach is to prevent them from being made in the first place, which is glutathione's role. Hydrogen peroxides have to be kept at a low, steady state in the body, and that is the job of glutathione.

By now you know that one of the most important jobs of antioxidants is to protect DNA, the genetic material within the cell, from oxidative damage. In this regard, glutathione not only functions as an antioxidant but goes one step further: Glutathione is also essential to prime DNA synthesis for cell replication. If DNA is damaged, there are enzymes that need to be activated to repair it, and that is one of glutathione's many jobs.

Glutathione is instrumental in the storage and transport of amino acids, the building blocks of protein. Amino acids cannot cross cell membranes on their own—they need to hitch a ride on special transport systems. Glutathione contains two amino acids, cysteine and methionine, which cross the cell membrane as part of the glutathione molecule, and then go their separate ways once they are in the cell.

Glutathione turns off the inflammatory response

Similar to other network antioxidants, glutathione is also a signaling molecule that turns on and turns off genes. In particular, glutathione is involved in regulating the pathway that activates genes that can cause chronic inflammation and lead to serious health problems such as arthritis, autoimmune diseases, and even cancer.

If your lungs are your Achilles' heel—if every cold you get turns into bronchitis or even pneumonia—you should be vigilant about maintaining your glutathione levels. Glutathione and associated enzymes are found in the lining of the lungs, and undoubtedly they are there for a good reason. With every breath you take, lung tissue is bombarded with high levels of both oxygen and pollutants. Glutathione, along with the other network antioxidants, can protect against oxidative damage from these environmental stressors. In fact, low levels of reduced glutathione (and higher than normal levels of oxidized glutathione) are typically found in the lungs of people with chronic respiratory ailments such as asthma.

Glutathione: the body's detoxifier

As I mentioned earlier, there are very high concentrations of glutathione in liver cells, for good reason. The liver, one of the body's largest internal organs, has numerous jobs and is vital for survival. The liver is involved in the production of bile, which is necessary for the breakdown of fat and storage of glycogen to fuel muscles, and the storage of fat-soluble vitamins A, D, and K. The liver also produces other important substances such as clotting factors, blood proteins, and thousands of different enzymes. One of the liver's most critical roles is detoxification of drugs and poisons that may be either ingested through food or drugs or produced by the body through normal metabolism.

The ability of the body to detoxify poisons is key to our survival. With every breath we take, and every meal we eat, we are exposed to thousands of potential toxins. Insecticides in food and water, cleaning fluids used at home and in industry, and even drugs that may be prescribed by your doctor could break down into substances in the body that can be dangerous. Fortunately, with the help of glutathione, our livers are usually able to handle this burden.

Glutathione is an essential part of the detoxification process. When glutathione encounters toxic compounds in the liver, it attaches onto them, and in a process called *S-conjugation,* makes the compound more water-soluble. That allows toxins to be flushed out through the kidneys.

A well-functioning liver is essential for good health, and when the liver does not function properly, it can lead to serious illness and death. There is a strong correlation between liver diseases such as cirrhosis (inflammation) of the liver and low levels of glutathione. In the chapter on lipoic acid, I described how lipoic acid is now being used successfully to treat liver disease. Since lipoic acid boosts glutathione levels, it could very well be that its positive effect on liver function is actually caused by its ability to increase glutathione.

Steroid hormones (such as estrogen and testosterone) and hormone-like compounds called prostaglandins are also broken down in the liver. Maintaining the right levels of hormones is critical for the proper functioning of the body. Some studies suggest that higher than normal levels of certain steroid hormones may increase the risk of developing hormone-sensitive cancers such as breast cancer. Glutathione plays a role in helping to control the levels of hormones and prostaglandins, just one of many examples of how this antioxidant safeguards our health.

Glutathione rejuvenates immune function

Immune function, in particular the effectiveness of T-cells (the body's primary disease-fighting cells), declines with age. When an animal is depleted of glutathione, its immune function declines dramatically. Not so coincidentally, in both illness and old age in humans, glutathione levels can drop precipitously. Numerous studies document glutathione's role in many different aspects of T-cell function, including the production of T-cells.

Recently researchers at the USDA Human Nutrition Research Center on Aging devised an experiment to test the effect of glutathione on both young and aging immune cells. Immune cells were removed from the blood of thirty-five- to forty-five-year-old men, and also sixty-five- to eighty-four-year-old men. The cells were placed in a test tube with very high glutathione concentrations, much higher than normally found in blood plasma. Interestingly, the glutathione did not have much effect on the immune cells of the younger participants, but there were significant changes in the immune cells of the older participants. In particular, the glutathione stimulated the production of interleukin 1 (IL-1), which is involved in inflammatory responses that are necessary to effectively fight against infection, and IL-2, which is involved in the growth of new immune cells. Indeed, glutathione also increased lymphocyte proliferation, which means the old immune cells were able to reproduce more rapidly. The net effect of glutathione supplementation was to give immune cells more ammunition to fight against foreign invaders.

Although glutathione supplementation did not appear to have any effect on the immune cells of younger people, glutathione depletion at any age will affect immune function, even among the most fit of athletes. In my laboratory, Dr. Kishor Gohil and I have shown that glutathione levels can be seriously depleted by strenuous physical activity. Vigorous exercise increases energy utilization, which increases the level of free radicals, which in turn can inhibit immune cells. Marathon runners frequently contract respiratory infections after a big race. This is no mere coincidence; it is caused by increased oxidative stress owing to the enormous physical strain they have put on their bodies, which leaves them more vulnerable to infection. This is why it is so important for athletes of any age to be careful about maintaining their antioxidant defenses.

Glutathione: an antiaging antioxidant

The free radical theory of aging first proposed by Denham Harman blames the aging process on cumulative damage to cells and tissues inflicted over many decades by exposure to free radicals. Several studies have suggested that levels of glutathione decline with age, and of course this idea has led to speculation that the drop in glutathione may exacerbate the aging process.

Boosting levels of specific antioxidants (such as vitamin E) can extend life in animals. In one experiment, researchers at the University of Louisville School of Medicine hypothesized that if the decline in glutathione was responsible for the aging process, then replenishing glutathione in older animals should help extend life. For their experiment, they selected the yellow fever mosquito, an excellent model for human aging for several reasons. First, the biochemical function of mosquitoes is quite similar to mammals; second, they are genetically easy to manipulate; and finally, they have a life span of only thirty days, which means the experiments can be performed quickly. In this particular experiment, mosquitoes were given NAC, which is known to boost glutathione 50 to 100 percent in the cells of mosquitoes. The result was that the mosquitoes with the elevated glutathione levels lived about 40 percent longer than normal.

In another study recently performed in Switzerland, researchers added high doses of NAC to the diet of fruit flies, which are also a wonderful model for human aging. The good news is that the NAC-supplemented fruit flies lived on average more than 16 percent longer than normal. The even better news is that NAC treatment actually extended the life span of fruit flies by more than 26 percent. What is particularly intriguing is that while it is not unusual for a substance to extend the life of an animal, it is highly unusual to extend the life span, that is, the uppermost life expectancy for a particular species.

Obviously, the prospect of mosquitoes or fruit flies living longer is not why I am so excited about these studies. The reality is that what's good for the mosquito or the fruit fly is often good for human beings as well. In fact, much of the exciting work in science that produced giant leaps forward often began with tiny organisms like mosquitoes and flies.

If boosting glutathione levels works as well in older humans as it does in insects, living to be 100 and beyond could become a reality for us in the next century. I believe that restoring the entire antioxidant network will have an even more profound effect on our health and longevity, and that the best approach is to keep the entire antioxidant network strong and fully charged.

Enhancing the power of the antioxidant network will enable us to keep our antioxidant advantage, which we need in order to defeat the forces that can age us prematurely and rob us of our health. One way we can enhance the antioxidant network is by increasing our intake of Antioxidant Boosters—substances that may or may not be antioxidants themselves but can have a profound effect on the antioxidant network.

In Part Three, I will discuss the major Antioxidant Boosters and how they can vastly extend the power of the antioxidant network.

Network

Boosters

9

The Flavonoids
The Healing Power of Plants—
Ginkgo Biloba and Pycnogenol

❋ Flavonoids improve memory and concentration and are used to treat attention deficit disorder.

❋ Flavonoids are powerful free radical scavengers that can boost the effectiveness of C in the antioxidant network.

❋ Flavonoids regulate nitric oxide, a potent free radical that is a regulator of blood flow.

❋ Flavonoids keep your heart healthy in three important ways: They prevent blood clots, protect against the oxidation of LDL cholesterol, and lower high blood pressure.

❋ Flavonoids improve sexual function in men.

❋ Flavonoids reduce inflammation and bolster immune function.

❋ *RDA:* None.

❋ *The Packer Plan:* Ginkgo biloba: 30 milligrams daily; Pycnogenol: 20 milligrams daily.

❋ *Sources:* Not produced in the body but found in abundance in plants, fruits and vegetables, and plant-based beverages. Best sources include tea leaves, oranges, citrus fruit, apples, onions, red grapes, berries, and pine bark.

Flavonoids are a group of more than 4,000 individual compounds that are found in plants, notably in the pigments of leaves, barks, rinds, seeds, and flowers. They are part of a larger group of molecules called *polyphenol compounds*. All flavonoids are antioxidants, but some are stronger antioxidants than others, depending on their molecular structure.

About fifty flavonoids are present in foods and beverages derived from plants, such as berries, tea, and wine. Although they are not network antioxidants, my laboratory has discovered that flavonoids interact with the network by regenerating vitamin C back to its active antioxidant form after it has quenched a free radical. This exciting discovery has broad implications not just for vitamin C, but for the entire antioxidant network. Boosting vitamin C also increases levels of vitamin E, which will provide protection for both the water-soluble and fat-soluble parts of the cell.

In particular, we have found that complex mixtures of flavonoids, such as those found in Pycnogenol (pine bark extract) and ginkgo biloba extract, are even more powerful than their individual components. Once again this shows that antioxidants are meant to work together, and in almost every circumstance, combinations of antioxidants have been proven to be more effective than single antioxidants. In addition to their role as network boosters, flavonoids have other jobs in the body that make them essential for optimal health.

Before we modern-day scientists take all the credit for discovering flavonoids, I must admit that we are not the first to explore the medicinal properties of these intriguing plants. In fact, in this respect, we have a lot of catching up to do. For more than 5,000 years, so-called medicine men, practitioners of herbal medicine, have been prescribing flavonoid compounds to treat a wide variety of ailments, from circulatory problems to skin conditions to inflammatory diseases. These early healers knew what we are just proving in the laboratory: flavonoids can be powerful medicine.

Although flavonoids are not produced in the body, they are not listed on the RDAs. In fact, until recently they were regarded as little more than food dye, and their 5,000-year history in traditional medicine was virtually ignored by all but a few researchers. In the 1960s, some physicians prescribed flavonoids to treat problems such as gum disease and circulatory disorders but were discouraged from doing so in the 1970s when the USDA issued a report dismissing flavonoids as worthless.

What a difference a decade or two make—today there are volumes of studies confirming that flavonoids are not just for plants but are powerful medicine for humans as well. For example, a now famous 1996 Dutch study of 522 men found that those who drank the most tea, a rich source of flavonoids, had a significantly lower risk of developing stroke than those who did not. Numerous studies have documented that people who drink red wine, which is particularly high in flavonoids, have much lower rates of heart disease than teetotalers. For example, even though the French eat foods that are laden with fat, such as butter and pâté, and smoking is a national hobby, heart disease is relatively rare. This so-called French Paradox is attributed to their relatively high intake of flavonoids through red wine as compared to consumption of wine in the United States. And literally hundreds of studies, many performed in my laboratory, show that flavonoids play an important role in the antioxidant network. Unfortunately, this new information is not yet reflected in the RDAs, and I doubt it will be in the near future.

Although they had been used for thousands of years, flavonoids were officially identified and isolated by Albert Szent-Györgyi, the Nobel Laureate who was the first to isolate vitamin C. Interestingly, Szent-Györgyi recognized that flavonoids had a synergistic relationship with vitamin C, which we confirmed more than sixty years later in our laboratory. In an article in *Nature,* the premier scientific journal, Szent-Györgyi noted: "Various chemical and clinical observations have led to the assumption that ascorbic acid is accompanied in the cell by a substance of similar important and related activity."

He called this substance "vitamin P." In the article, Szent-Györgyi reported that he had found a cure for a problem characterized by increased fragility of the capillary wall. Although vitamin C alone had been ineffective, when combined with extracts of Hungarian red pepper or lemon juice, which contained flavonoids, the condition cleared up.

My work has focused primarily on two particularly fascinating flavonoid-containing plant extract preparations that are deeply rooted in traditional medicine, yet hold great promise as treatments for many modern ailments. The first is ginkgo biloba (ginkgo for short), derived from the leaves of the ginkgo tree, one of the oldest trees on Earth. The second is Pycnogenol, a patented extract from French maritime pine bark that contains about forty different antioxidant flavonoids. Ginkgo and Pycnogenol are similar in many of the roles they play in the body, yet as you will see, each is unique. Both are available in capsule form at health food stores and pharmacies.

Before I review the specific benefits offered by these special booster antioxidants, I would like to tell you about the third and perhaps most important component of the flavonoid story. It is not about another antioxidant; rather it is about the free radical that antioxidant flavonoids help to control—nitric oxide.

Flavonoids and the nitric oxide connection

Nitric oxide is a colorless gas produced by many different cells in the body, from endothelial cells on the walls of arteries to the neurons in the brain to the disease-fighting cells of the immune system. I call nitric oxide the Jekyll and Hyde of molecules because it has a split personality: depending on the situation, it can be very good or very bad.

Until recently, nitric oxide was considered to be nothing but bad. This ubiquitous free radical was found in all the wrong places, including smog, automobile exhaust, and cigarette smoke. Not only was it blamed for destroying the ozone layer, it was widely believed to be a potent carcinogen. In the late 1980s, scientists began to notice that nitric oxide appeared to be a key player in many essential bodily functions. Paradoxically, this "good" free radical could be dangerous under the wrong conditions, but beneficial under the right conditions.

Nitric oxide plays several important roles in the body:

* Nitric oxide is an important signaling molecule that turns genes on and off.

* By controlling the muscular tone of blood vessels, nitric oxide regulates circulation and normalizes blood flow.

* Nitric oxide modulates communication between brain cells and is instrumental in helping us concentrate and learn new information, and also in maintaining memory.

* When produced by immune cells, nitric oxide fights infection, kills tumor cells, and promotes wound healing.

* Nitric oxide is essential for perceiving pleasure and pain, and it helps translate sexual excitement into penile erections.

* Nitric oxide aids in digestion of food by helping to control gastric movements.

But nitric oxide can be very destructive under other circumstances:

* It restricts blood flow, contributing to heart disease and stroke.

* When produced in excess by immune cells, nitric oxide can trigger chronic inflammation, which can cause arthritis, colitis, inflammatory bowel disease, and possibly even cancer.

* It promotes production of more free radicals.

* In the brain it can hamper mental function and cause memory loss and brain aging.

When nitric oxide encounters the superoxide free radical, it goes from bad to worse. It becomes a peroxynitrite, which destroys antioxidants like glutathione, flavonoids, and vitamin E and damages proteins.

The question is, why does good nitric oxide go bad? As long as it is produced in the right amount, nitric oxide will remain friendly, but if it is overproduced, the effect can be toxic. We have found that flavonoid antioxidants like ginkgo and Pycnogenol can regulate nitric oxide, helping to maintain the optimal level of this free radical. As you will see, each of these flavonoids can do this and much more.

Ginkgo biloba

The ginkgo is of Stone Age origin, making it one of the oldest living trees on the planet. Once ubiquitous in North America and Europe, it was destroyed during the Ice Age everywhere on Earth except in China, where it still lives and thrives. It was brought to America in 1784 and is now one of the most common trees in the United States.

Ginkgo is a strong, hardy tree that can grow as tall as 122 feet and 4 feet in diameter. It is well known for its longevity: some ginkgos have lived to be 1,000 years old. Undoubtedly, ancient healers took note of the strength and vigor of the ginkgo and concluded that it could be beneficial to humans. The leaves and fruit of the ginkgo have been used as a medicinal treatment in China since 2800 B.C., primarily for problems related to brain function, heart disease, and other circulatory disorders.

As more and more Americans turn to traditional medicine, ginkgo has become one of the most popular supplements to date. Ginkgo is primarily being touted as a memory-enhancing herb, and as I will explain, there is some scientific basis to this claim. In Germany and France ginkgo is sold as a prescription drug; it is one of the most widely prescribed medications in the world. In the United States, ginkgo is considered a supplemental herb and is sold over-the-counter.

I first became interested in ginkgo because I suspected that much of its reputed benefits were derived from its antioxidant action, specifically its role as a modulator of nitric oxide production. We tested ginkgo extract against several common free radicals, and it passed with flying colors. Not only did it inhibit the action of nitric oxide, but it also quenched superoxide and the hydroxyl radical, two powerful and potentially dangerous free radicals.

It became apparent that nature had equipped this ancient tree with the tools it needed for a long, healthy life, and that perhaps we could also benefit from it.

Flavonoids promote good circulation

When healers first prescribed ginkgo for circulatory problems, they could only have guessed what we can now prove in the laboratory: ginkgo is good for the heart.

In the Packer Lab, we have shown that ginkgo extract can prevent the oxidation of low-density lipoproteins (or LDL cholesterol).

We have also shown that ginkgo can speed up recovery after a heart attack. We tested ginkgo in a simulated heart attack using what is called the Langendorff beating-heart model. We then reperfused the beating hearts with a solution that did not contain oxygen, thus inducing a heart attack. After forty minutes, we changed solutions, this time using one that contained oxygen. Under these circumstances, only 20 to 25 percent of the hearts will recover, that is, continue beating normally. The rest will suffer serious damage, including irreparable destruction of heart muscle. Eventually, the hearts will die. When we added ginkgo to the reperfusion solution, however, the rate of recovery soared to 65 percent, and there was also a significant reduction in tissue damage. This experiment showed that ginkgo extract can rescue a dying heart, enabling it to survive an otherwise lethal heart attack.

Flavonoids: treatment for impotence

Good circulation is not only important for heart health but is essential for the functioning of every system, including the reproductive system. There are two primary ways that ginkgo can help to preserve and perhaps even enhance sexual function in men.

First, ginkgo can help to prevent the leading cause of male impotence—atherosclerosis. It may surprise you to learn that about half of the cases of male impotence are not caused by hormonal or psychological problems, but by clogged arteries. In order to maintain an erection, blood must flow freely to the penis. If the blood flow becomes narrowed or clogged because of atherosclerosis, the blood supply will be impaired.

Nitric oxide is also critical in translating sexual excitement into penile erection. In the brain, a hormone called *oxytocin* induces the synthesis of an enzyme that turns on the production of nitric oxide. When this happens, the parasympathetic nervous system is activated. At the nerve endings, the nitric oxide–producing enzyme is induced, leading to a localized production of nitric oxide. This stimulates the relaxation of smooth muscles, allowing the arteries supplying blood to the penis to dilate. Nitric oxide is also produced by endothelial cells lining the blood vessels in the penis, which are constantly producing nitric oxide at a very low level. As I noted earlier, ginkgo as well as other flavonoids can help to maintain the right balance of nitric oxide in the body, which will help improve sexual function. (Viagra, the medication that helps certain kinds of male impotence, works indirectly by stimulating nitric oxide metabolism.)

There has been at least one study testing the effect of ginkgo on impotent men, and the results have been noteworthy. In the study, reported in the *Journal of Urology*, fifty impotent men were given 240 milligrams of ginkgo extract daily for nine months. Some of the men were also given injections of a drug called papaverine, a muscle stimulant that can boost erections. The ginkgo supplements alone greatly improved erections in both groups of men, whether or not they had taken the papaverine injections. Ginkgo did not work overnight, but it did work reasonably well: It took up to eight weeks for the men to first begin to see an improvement, and by six months of therapy, half of the patients had regained potency.

Flavonoids are a brain booster

Of all of its potential uses, ginkgo's primary claim to fame is as a brain booster. In Germany and France, ginkgo is commonly prescribed for mental problems that are often caused by poor circulation to the brain, such as difficulty concentrating, poor memory, confusion, depression, and anxiety. There have been numerous European studies performed on ginkgo and many have reported positive effects in terms of memory and acuity. I'm not suggesting that ginkgo is going to turn you into a rocket scientist, but given all we know about ginkgo's effect on both nitric oxide metabolism and circulation, it makes sense that it may offer benefits in enhancing memory.

Recently, ginkgo extract was tested on patients suffering from dementia (caused by either stroke or Alzheimer's disease) with positive results. In the study, which was performed at the New York Institute for Medical Research, 327 patients with dementia were randomly assigned to take a 120-milligram capsule of ginkgo extract daily or a placebo. Only 137 patients actually completed the study, and out of that group, about 30 percent of those taking ginkgo showed better results on tests of reasoning, memory, and behavior than the placebo users. The effects of ginkgo were described as "modest" by the researchers conducting the study, but since there are few drugs that have any impact at all in cases of dementia, even this limited positive result generated much excitement and publicity. I don't believe that ginkgo alone is going to prove to be the magic bullet for Alzheimer's disease, but I do believe that the antioxidant network and its boosters will be proven to play a role in slowing down the progression of this disease.

Flavonoids are a natural anti-inflammatory

When the immune system detects danger, it responds by sending cells to the area of injury. Special immune cells called *macrophages* produce cell adhesion molecule proteins that are important because they help immune cells attach themselves to foreign invaders and thereby defeat them. Cell adhesion molecule proteins are an important part of the healing process, but excessive amounts of cell adhesion molecule proteins can be dangerous and are a contributing factor to inflammatory diseases such as rheumatoid arthritis and even cancer. In test tube studies, we have shown that ginkgo can inhibit the overproduction of cell adhesion molecule proteins in human macrophages, an indication that it would work the same way in the human body.

Our work with ginkgo may have just begun, but based on what we have already learned, I have no doubt that ginkgo will prove to be an important addition to the antioxidant family.

Pycnogenol: the pine bark miracle

Pine bark is another flavonoid mixture that has also been used for thousands of years by traditional healers but is just being discovered by modern scientists. Pycnogenol is the registered trademark name for a mix of about forty different antioxidants that are extracted from the bark of the French maritime pine tree *(Pinus maritima).* Since ancient times, pine bark has been used as both a source of food and medicine. Hippocrates (400 B.C.), credited with being the father of modern medicine, prescribed pine bark for inflammatory disorders. The pounded inner pulp of the pine bark was used on inflamed wounds, sores, and ulcers. It was also made into a cough medicine. Modern-day Laplanders, who must suffer through the brutally cold northern winters, grind pine bark into flour and make it into bread. This makes a lot of sense—as I will explain, we have learned that compounds in pine bark can enhance immune function and therefore offered protection against winter colds and flus. (I've sampled pine bark bread, and it tastes better than it sounds.)

The particular species of pine bark used in Pycnogenol has a fascinating history that has only recently been brought to light. In 1535, French explorer and navigator Jacques Cartier was sailing up what is now known as the Saint Lawrence River in Canada. It was the dead of winter, and when the river froze, his ship was stranded. Lacking fresh fruits and vegetables, Cartier's crew quickly fell victim to what we now know is scurvy, caused by severe vitamin C deficiency. The telltale symptoms included fatigue, bleeding gums, skin hemorrhages, fragile bones, erratic behavior, and extreme irritability. More than twenty-five sailors

died before the crew was rescued by friendly Quebec Indians who recommended that they drink a tea made from the bark of native pine
trees. Miraculously, after drinking the tea, and rubbing it on their
swollen, inflamed bodies, the crew was cured within a week. Cartier
wrote about his experiences in a book called *Voyages au Canada,* which
remained unnoticed until by chance it was read by Canadian scientist
Jacques Masquelier in the 1960s, who found it at the University of
Quebec library. Coincidentally, Masquelier was doing research on
flavonoids.

Masquelier found Cartier's story both puzzling and intriguing. He
knew that pine needles had only a minute quantity of vitamin C—
certainly not enough to cure scurvy—and pine bark had none. Why did
the crew recover after drinking the tea? There was only one logical
explanation: Masquelier concluded that pine bark must contain
flavonoids that greatly enhanced the effect of the tiny amount of vitamin C found in the pine needles. He set out to prove his theory and,
in the process, discovered that the particular species of pine bark used
by Cartier contained significant amounts of potent antioxidant substances called *proanthocyanidins* (known as OPCs for short). In 1987,
Masquelier was granted a U.S. patent for Pycnogenol.

As part of my antioxidant research, I became aware of Masquelier's
work. Since Pycnogenol boosted vitamin C, I became intrigued by the
possibility that Pycnogenol's effect may be caused by its ability to recycle vitamin C in the network. In other words, even though Pycnogenol
was not a network antioxidant, I suspected that it could interact with
the network in positive ways. I was right. In the test tube, we found that
Pycnogenol extends the lifetime of vitamin C, a sign that it is recycling
C back to its antioxidant form.

Our research team has looked at the antioxidant power of several
extracts from fruits and vegetables including ginkgo, green tea, and
other flavonoids, all of which boosted C, but none worked as well as
Pycnogenol. We have also found that Pycnogenol can boost the body's
production of other antioxidants, such as vitamin E and glutathione,
further increasing cell defenses against free radical attack.

In fact, of all the natural compounds tested in my laboratory for
antioxidant activity, Pycnogenol is the strongest. We found that
Pycnogenol could quench superoxide, nitric oxide, and the hydroxyl
radical. This is extremely important. Of all the free radicals formed in

the body, the hydroxyl radical is the most dangerous because it can directly attack DNA.

Pycnogenol's antioxidant activity was identified more than twenty years ago, but we have only learned about its incredible power, and in particular, its ability to control nitric oxide. I would like to share with you some of the most interesting scientific findings on Pycnogenol so that you can understand why I am so excited about this intriguing flavonoid.

Flavonoids protect against heart disease

Since the 1930s, scientists have known that flavonoids enhanced the activity of vitamin C, which is essential for the production of mature collagen that lines the walls of capillaries, the body's smallest blood vessels. Although capillaries are very small, they are very important in that they form the foundation of the body's cardiovascular system. Capillary walls must be strong, yet flexible enough to allow blood to flow freely. When capillaries become weak, they can rupture or block the flow of blood. A person who bruises very easily has very weak capillary walls. Weak capillaries can also become leaky and can lead to edema, which most people know as fluid retention or swelling. Pycnogenol improves microcirculation by reinforcing capillary walls, making them more resilient.

There's yet another way that Pycnogenol may protect against cardiovascular disease. Pycnogenol protects against platelet aggregation, the first step in the formation of blood clots. In humans, Pycnogenol inhibited platelet aggregation in smokers in response to adrenaline. Blood clots are dangerous because they can lead to heart attack and stroke. As many of you may know, doctors frequently recommend that their patients take aspirin to prevent blood clots. Although aspirin works well for this purpose, it can also cause potentially dangerous side effects such as prolonged bleeding, gastrointestinal distress, or even bleeding ulcers.

The good news is that Pycnogenol works even better than aspirin in terms of controlling platelet aggregation, but without the unwanted side effects associated with aspirin. Pycnogenol reduced human smoking-induced platelet aggregation to the same extent as a five-times-higher dose of aspirin.

Flavonoids strengthen the immune function

A strong immune system is the cornerstone of good health: if your immune system is weak, it will eventually affect the other systems of your body. Pycnogenol can help fortify your immune system in several important ways. First, by increasing the activity of vitamin C, another important immune booster, Pycnogenol gives the immune system more ammunition to fight against infection. Second, our experiments have shown that Pycnogenol prevents free radical damage to macrophages, a type of white blood cell that generates the free radical nitric oxide to destroy bacteria, viruses, and host parasites. Here is another example of how free radicals are necessary enemies. We need them to kill off foreign invaders, but if they are overproduced, they will turn on their host and damage the macrophages.

In cell culture studies, we used bacterial toxins to trigger the release of nitric oxide from macrophages. As expected, large amounts of the nitric oxide radicals started killing off the macrophages themselves! If this was happening inside a human being, it would be fair to assume that his or her ability to fight infection would be impaired. However, when we added Pycnogenol to the mix, nitric oxide production decreased significantly, and macrophages were unharmed and allowed to continue their disease-fighting activity.

Researchers at the University of Arizona confirm that Pycnogenol has an immune-enhancing effect not just in cell cultures, but in animals. Under the direction of Ronald Watson, Ph.D., researchers tested Pycnogenol in a mouse model of an HIV-like virus and alcoholism, two conditions that can compromise normal immune function. Pycnogenol boosted immune function in the immune-damaged mice by increasing production of interleukin-2, which promotes the activity of T-cells and lymphocytes and enables the body to fight more effectively against infection. In healthy mice, Pycnogenol stimulates natural killer cells (NK-cells), which help the body ward off cancer. NK-cells are constantly monitoring our bodies for signs of abnormal growth that could result in cancer. When NK-cells identify abnormally reproducing cells, they attack them. If Pycnogenol has a similar effect in humans, it could offer powerful protection against many different types of cancer.

Flavonoids and chronic fatigue syndrome

For centuries, healers have used pine bark to treat inflammatory disorders such as rheumatoid arthritis, a condition in which the cells of the immune system attack the body's own tissue, destroying the joint cartilage. Free radicals are believed to be a major factor in the progression of rheumatoid arthritis and other inflammatory diseases. Several antioxidants, including Pycnogenol and vitamins C and E, can relieve some of the disease's symptoms, such as pain and swelling.

Recently, researchers have investigated whether Pycnogenol would be an effective treatment for another chronic inflammatory condition for which there is no treatment—chronic fatigue syndrome (CFS). CFS produces symptoms similar to rheumatoid arthritis but is even more complicated to treat. CFS is characterized as an unexplained debilitating fatigue that lasts for six months or longer and is not caused by any underlying physical problem. In addition to exhaustion, people with CFS often complain of arthritic-type muscle and joint pain, swollen glands, headache, depression, and confusion. Although anti-inflammatory drugs and antidepressants are often prescribed for this problem, there is no cure, and all of these drugs can cause unpleasant side effects. In fact, the long-term use of anti-inflammatory medications can lead to bleeding ulcers and other serious gastrointestinal problems. Pycnogenol may offer a ray of hope to CFS patients.

According to researcher Anthony W. Martin, D.C., Ph.D., a chiropractor and health consultant on the faculty of LaSalle University in Canada, many CFS patients report good results with Pycnogenol, and in particular claim that it helps to relieve the often debilitating muscle pain that interferes with daily activities. Pycnogenol's positive effect on CFS is probably caused by its ability to improve circulation, which sends more blood to muscles, which in turn would result in a reduction in pain. In addition, Pycnogenol's antioxidant activity could help relieve some of the inflammation that could be contributing to the general discomfort experienced by CFS sufferers. Since Pycnogenol is completely safe and offers other benefits, it makes sense for people with chronic fatigue syndome to see if it works for them.

Flavonoids slow down aging

One of the most exciting experiments performed at the Packer Lab is one involving Pycnogenol in a model of cell death that mimics the aging process. As we age, cells begin to die in a process known as *apoptosis*. Sometimes it is to our benefit for cells to die, as in the case of cancer cells that would spread if they were allowed to live. However, as we age, there is a tendency for healthy cells to begin to die, which can seriously interfere with the functioning of important organs. For example, aging is typically associated with a marked decline in brain cells, which can result in a loss of memory, and even more serious conditions such as Alzheimer's and Parkinson's disease.

In our study, we grew brain cells in culture and exposed them to high levels of glutamate, an amino acid that is naturally produced by the body and is used as a neurotransmitter by the brain cells. At normal levels, glutamate is good, but in excess, it can destroy glutathione and trigger apoptosis. In fact, there are high levels of glutamate in the brain cells of people with Alzheimer's disease, brain injuries, AIDS, and cancer. Brain cells exposed to glutamate will begin to die rapidly. However, when we added Pycnogenol to the cell culture, the brain cells did not die. They continued to function normally. Although this experiment was performed outside of the body, it strongly suggests that Pycnogenol may slow down or even prevent cell death from occurring inside the body, particularly in vulnerable areas like the brain.

Flavonoids and attention-deficit hyperactivity disorder

When experiments in my laboratory first revealed that Pycnogenol had a modulating effect on nitric oxide, I hypothesized that it could be a potential treatment for attention-deficit hyperactivity disorder (ADHD), a condition that is characterized by the inability to concentrate, impulsivity, and hyperactivity. No one knows the cause of ADHD, but at least one major study showed that people with ADHD have less blood flow directed to the part of the brain that helps to organize behavior. Since nitric oxide is instrumental in circulation, it seemed probable that an imbalance of nitric oxide could be at the root of this common problem.

As many as 9 percent of all school-aged youngsters may have some form of ADHD, which often makes it extremely difficult for them to function well in a classroom. ADHD can also affect adults—as many as 60 percent of all childhood cases persist into adulthood. The standard drug therapy for ADHD is methylphenidate (Ritalin), a central nervous system stimulant. Although it is effective in terms of helping many children and adults with ADHD, in some people it can cause unpleasant side effects, including insomnia, nervousness, dizziness, and headaches.

Although Ritalin is both safe and effective, many parents are reluctant to give any prescription drug to their children over a long time and have sought a natural alternative. Since ADHD was reported to be linked to abnormal blood circulation, several innovative physicians in the United States and Europe have tried Pycnogenol on their ADHD patients. To date, there are numerous anecdotal reports that Pycnogenol works extremely well for many people with this problem.

Julie Paull, Ph.D., and Steven Tenenbaum, Ph.D., licensed psychologists at the Attention Deficit Center in St. Louis, are conducting the first human clinical trial of adults ages eighteen to sixty-five to determine whether Pycnogenol is an effective treatment for this problem. Dr. Paull suffers from one form of ADHD herself, called the predominantly inattentive type. Contrary to popular belief, all people with ADHD are not necessarily overactive; in fact, some may appear to be passive and lethargic. What they have in common with other ADHD people is that they typically have difficulty focusing and easily run out of mental stamina.

Often, this more subtle form of ADHD goes undetected, as was the case with Dr. Paull, who recognized she had a problem but didn't precisely know what it was. Although she was high functioning and did well at school, she was aware that it took an enormous amount of energy for her to maintain her concentration. In fact, her professors would often comment that although she was bright and was wonderful with abstract reasoning, she appeared to have difficulty keeping track of details. Only when she began working in an ADHD clinic as a graduate student did Dr. Paull recognize her ADHD and seek help. Dr. Paull first tried Ritalin and found it somewhat helpful, but she didn't like the side effects, which included a twitch. She then switched to a tricyclic antidepressant, which is the second choice of conventional medicine for treating ADHD symptoms. Although the drug helped a bit, it did not improve her ability to focus. She felt she had no other alternative.

Dr. Paull heard about Pycnogenol from a patient who from anecdotal reports on the Internet knew that it was being used for ADHD. After doing some additional research, Dr. Paull was impressed enough by what she had learned to try Pycnogenol herself, adding it to her treatment regimen.

The results were amazing. "Five days later, I noticed a huge difference," Dr. Paull recalled. "Some of my patients have likened it to putting on a pair of glasses—suddenly everything comes into focus. It has given me a clarity of thought that I did not have before." In particular, Dr. Paull noticed that Pycnogenol has helped her better organize her thoughts, which has greatly increased her productivity. Although Pycnogenol alone may relieve ADHD symptoms in many people, for others it will work best when used along with other therapies.

The more we learn about antioxidants and free radicals, the more apparent it becomes that achieving the antioxidant advantage is the key to maintaining optimal physical and mental function. It is impossible to have one without the other. I am not surprised that two flavonoids—ginkgo biloba and Pycnogenol—are being used to treat problems related to memory, learning, and behavior. As we expand our definition of antioxidant, we are learning that these remarkable natural substances do far more than we imagined, and they will continue to capture our imagination for many years to come.

10

The Controversial Carotenoids

Alpha Carotene, Beta Carotene, Cryptoxanthin, Lutein, Lycopene, and Zeaxanthin

* Increased intake of carotenoid-rich foods and high blood levels of carotenoids offer powerful protection against many different types of cancer. One carotenoid in particular, lycopene, has been associated with lower rates of prostate cancer.

* Two carotenoids found in the eye, lutein and zeaxanthin, are associated with a decreased risk of macular degeneration and cataracts.

* Beta carotene can boost immune function in older people, but mixed carotenoids may do it better.

* A carotenoid-rich diet may reduce the risk of heart disease.

* *RDA:* There is no RDA for carotenoids.

* *The Packer Plan:* Most people can get enough carotenoids through their diet by eating three orange and yellow fruits and vegetables and two dark green leafy vegetables daily. If you are

at very high risk of developing heart disease or cancer, add two extra fruits or vegetables to your daily diet.

❋ *Supplements:* If you do not eat adequate amounts of carotenoid-rich foods, consider taking a mixed carotenoid supplement.

❋ *Caution:* Smokers should not take any carotenoid supplements but should eat a diet rich in fruits and vegetables.

❋ *Sources:* Brightly colored fruits and vegetables are the best sources of carotenoids.

Carotenoids are natural pigments found in both plants and animals. They are produced by bacteria, algae, fungi, and plants, but humans and animals get them through food.

There are more than 700 different carotenoids in nature, but only about 60 are found in food. The typical North American diet includes less than a dozen carotenoids. Researchers have focused primarily on six: alpha carotene, beta carotene, cryptoxanthin, lutein, lycopene, and zeaxanthin. Fruits and vegetables rich in carotenoids are known for their bright colors, ranging from brilliant yellow, red, and orange to purple and dark green.

Carotenoids are concentrated in the light-collecting centers of plants that are involved in photosynthesis and exposed to high levels of oxygen. Singlet oxygen, a highly reactive form of oxygen, is produced by photosynthesis. Although singlet oxygen is not a free radical itself, it promotes the formation of free radicals. Were it not for carotenoids, chlorophyll in leaves would be immediately bleached and destroyed by exposure to sunlight.

Carotenoids are unique in that some of them are converted into vitamin A in the body. Of all the carotenoids in our diet, only alpha carotene, beta carotene, and cryptoxanthin are converted into vitamin A.

Vitamin A is a fat-soluble vitamin that can be an antioxidant, but doesn't necessarily function as one in the body. Present in the rods and cones of the eye, vitamin A is responsible for color and black-and-white vision. In the body, vitamin A is converted into retinoic acid, which is an important molecule for activating genes.

Vitamin A is perhaps best known as a vitamin for healthy skin, and in particular, for its ability to protect against skin cancer. In a spectacular experiment performed in 1971 by Dr. Raymond Shamberger of the

Cleveland Clinic, a potent carcinogen was applied to the skin of mice. Under normal conditions, most of the mice would quickly develop skin cancer. When vitamin A was added to the carcinogen, however, it decreased the number of tumors by a remarkable 76 percent. This breakthrough led to a boon in vitamin A–derivative compounds used externally and internally to treat skin cancer.

Vitamin A–based skin-care products (such as Retin-A and retinoic acid) are also used to treat acne and signs of skin aging, such as sun spots and wrinkles. Used externally, vitamin A can help reduce the appearance of wrinkles by accelerating cell turnover and boosting the production of collagen.

Initially carotenoids were considered important only because they were precursors to vitamin A. It is now believed that individual carotenoids may play a role in the body that is unrelated to vitamin A.

Of all the antioxidants that I have reviewed in this book, carotenoids are by far the most controversial. For one thing, we're not sure they are true antioxidants. In the test tube, several carotenoids have exhibited strong antioxidant activity, but we have yet been able to prove that they act the same way in the human body. As far as we know, carotenoids are not part of the antioxidant network. If, however, they do function as antioxidants in humans—which they very well might—they could help the network by quenching free radicals, thereby reducing the workload for the network antioxidants.

What is not controversial is that numerous studies confirm that people who eat foods rich in carotenoids are significantly less likely to die of cancer than those who don't. Other studies have documented that people who have lower blood levels of certain carotenoids are more likely to develop cancer and heart disease as well as many other degenerative diseases than those with higher levels. However, these kinds of studies raise the question of whether it is an individual carotenoid, many different carotenoids, or even another substance such as fiber, which is also found in fruits and vegetables, that could be protective against disease.

When it comes to carotenoids, there are often more questions than answers. Beta carotene is the most abundant carotenoid in our diet and has become the focus of intense scientific scrutiny. It is also the most controversial of the carotenoids, for good reason.

The rise and fall of beta carotene

Beta carotene first captured the attention of the public after several studies linked a low intake of vitamin A and beta carotene–rich foods in the diet and low blood levels of both with an increased risk of getting cancer. (Because beta carotene was primarily known for its vitamin A activity, the early research lumped the two together.) Smokers had particularly low levels of vitamin A, and since smokers are at a substantially increased risk of getting many different types of cancer, it seemed reasonable to conclude that low levels of beta carotene may be responsible.

An abundance of animal studies seemed to reinforce the view that either beta carotene and/or vitamin A was protective against cancer. Beta carotene and vitamin A passed all the usual tests with flying colors. Mice injected with breast cancer cells had a much lower incidence of growing tumors if they were pretreated with vitamin A. In tissue culture studies, either vitamin A or beta carotene could inhibit the action of many different carcinogens. Animals that received transplanted tumors and were given vitamin A or beta carotene were much less likely to develop cancer than those that were not treated with vitamin A.

Then came the famous Westinghouse Electric study in which researchers traced the beta carotene intake of men over a nineteen-year period. At the study's conclusion, the researchers reported that among men who smoked, those who consumed the highest amounts of beta carotene had a significantly lower risk of developing lung cancer than those who had the lowest. In fact, the study came to the astonishing conclusion that smokers with the highest beta carotene intake from food had a similar risk of developing lung cancer as nonsmokers.

There was even more good news appearing in the scientific journals about beta carotene. Notably, studies showed that people who ate more fruits and vegetables—which are loaded with beta carotene—were much less likely to get heart disease.

By the early 1980s, beta carotene was touted as the hot cancer-fighting, heart-healthy supplement and quickly became a best-seller.

The only problem was that there was still no evidence that taking beta carotene supplements would actually help to prevent either heart disease or cancer in humans. Several studies were designed to answer this question. In one famous Finnish study a group of 29,133 male smokers were given either 20 milligrams of beta carotene a day or a placebo. Surprisingly, the men who took beta carotene had a slightly *increased* incidence of death from lung cancer. At first, this study was dismissed as a statistical fluke, but two other studies shed serious doubt on the ability of beta carotene supplements to protect smokers.

The Beta Carotene and Retinol Efficacy Trial, or CARET study, tested either a low dose of beta carotene or 25,000 I.U. of vitamin A on men and women who had a high risk of developing lung cancer—they had a history of exposure to asbestos, a known carcinogen, and many were heavy smokers. In the study involving more than 18,000 people, participants were given either beta carotene (30 milligrams daily), vitamin A, both, or a placebo. Much to the shock and dismay of the researchers, the people taking beta carotene with vitamin A had a 28 percent *higher* rate of mortality from lung cancer compared to the placebo group, and a general 17 percent *increase* in mortality. The results were so devastating that the study was discontinued twenty-one months ahead of schedule.

In yet another disappointing study, more than 22,000 physicians taking part in the Physicians' Health Study were either assigned to take 50 milligrams of beta carotene daily or a placebo to determine if it would reduce their risk of developing heart disease. Although numerous studies had suggested that people who ate the most beta carotene–rich foods had the lowest risk of heart disease, the beta carotene supplements did not appear to make any difference.

So what do all these statistics mean? First, it's important to remember that when beta carotene is obtained through food, it is also taken in combination with other carotenoids and phytochemicals, any or all of which could be responsible for the protective effect reported in earlier studies.

Second, critics of these studies argue that the participants were given a synthetic version of beta carotene that was not identical to the beta carotene found in food, or best used by the body. They contend that natural forms of beta carotene derived from plant sources would not produce the same ill effects. Whether this is true remains to be seen.

I have my own opinion—I believe that the CARET study may have been ill-conceived. The participants in the CARET study were walking time bombs: exposure to asbestos, particularly when combined with smoking (and in many cases, high alcohol consumption), is particularly lethal. It may simply have been too late to make a difference for this group.

I also believe that in some cases, the supplementation may have simply accelerated cancers that were already there. Here's why. In the body, beta carotene is broken down to make shorter chain compounds (like vitamin A and related retinols) that have very precise functions, and some abnormal compounds that may have unusual functions. These abnormal compounds are found in tiny concentrations and are usually harmless to most people. When combined with cigarette smoke or asbestos in the lung, however, these abnormal compounds may have promoted the growth of malignant cells. The moral of this tale is that if you smoke and/or have been exposed to asbestos, you should not take supplementary beta carotene. Since carotenoids obtained through food do not appear to increase cancer rates among smokers, and in fact may decrease it, it is also advisable to eat ample amounts of fresh fruits and vegetables.

What about nonsmokers? Should they take beta carotene? There is absolutely no evidence that even high doses of beta carotene supplements can cause any harm. The question is, do they help? I believe that if you do take a carotenoid supplement, it should be in the form of mixed carotenoids, which contain several different carotenoids that are normally found in food. This is the way the body is accustomed to handling carotenoids from food and is a more natural approach than simply taking one carotenoid.

Since the negative press on beta carotene, there have been some positive findings, notably on beta carotene's effect on immune function in older people. Dr. Michelle Santos of the USDA Human Nutrition Center on Aging recently reported that long-term supplementation of 50 milligrams of beta carotene daily for men between the ages of sixty-five and eighty-six resulted in stronger immune cell activity similar to what is seen in men twenty years their junior. In particular, there was a dramatic increase in natural killer (NK) cell activity, which is significant because these cells fight cancer. NK cells are constantly monitoring our bodies for signs of abnormal cell growth that could result in cancer. When they detect abnormal cells, they attack before the cells can spread. Recently, a small study involving mixed carotenoids administered to women showed that they bolstered immune function even better than beta carotene supplements.

There is some evidence, but not yet solid proof, that each of the carotenoids found in food may offer unique benefits. For example, some studies suggest that alpha carotene, found in carrots and pumpkin, may have an even stronger protective effect against cancer than beta carotene. It worked extremely well in preventing carcinogen-induced cancers in laboratory animals and in test tube studies, but whether it works the same way in humans remains to be seen.

Another carotenoid, cryptoxanthin, which is found in papayas, peaches, tangerines, and oranges, may protect against cervical cancer. A 1993 study revealed that cancer-free women had significantly higher levels of this carotenoid than those who had cervical cancer. Of course, the weakness in studies such as these is that cryptoxanthin-rich foods also contain other beneficial phytochemicals that could have a protective effect.

The science here is soft, and there are no easy or certain answers.

Pizza is an antioxidant: lycopene

Lycopene is the carotenoid that gives tomatoes their bright red color. It may also help protect against one of the most common cancers among men—prostate cancer.

The prostate is a small, walnut-size gland located between the penis and the bladder, above the rectum. The prostate produces semen, the fluid that carries sperm. Next to skin cancer, prostate cancer is the most common type of cancer to strike men. More than 200,000 new cases are diagnosed each year, and about 40,000 men die annually of this disease. Most new cases of prostate cancer strike men over age fifty-five: the average age of onset is seventy, so it is a disease associated with aging.

As with other cancers, diet appears to play a role in helping to prevent prostate cancer. In a six-year study of 48,000 male physicians conducted by Dr. Edward Giovanucci at Harvard Medical School, researchers found that men who consumed tomatoes, tomato sauce, or pizza more than twice a week showed a reduced risk of prostate cancer of 21 to 34 percent as opposed to those who did not eat these foods. All of these foods are rich in lycopene, the most prevalent carotenoid in human blood plasma. Interestingly, pizza was the food that seemed to offer the most protection. Researchers suspect that lycopene may be better absorbed when cooked with fat, such as the oil and cheese in pizza. Fresh tomato is not as good a source of lycopene.

Although it has not yet been proven, lycopene may function as an antioxidant in the body. In fact, test tube studies have shown that lycopene is a stronger antioxidant than beta carotene. There is other evidence that lycopene's protective action may extend beyond the prostate. Researchers at Ben Gurion University and Seroka Medical Center in Israel showed in the test tube that lycopene inhibited the growth of cancer cells from the breast, lung, and endothelial tissue. Lycopene can also thwart the growth of cancerous tumors in animals fed known carcinogens, which strongly suggests that it could have the same effect in humans.

Most researchers agree, however, that it is premature to advise men to take lycopene supplements, since we are not certain whether it is the lycopene alone, or lycopene combined with other nutrients in tomato, that protects against cancer. It is wise, however, for men to include more tomato-based products in their diet. Although the research has focused on lycopene, it is possible that the anticancer effects attributed to lycopene may be derived from another substance or substances in tomatoes that have not yet been identified. If you don't like tomatoes, lycopene is present in smaller amounts in guava, pink grapefruit, and watermelon.

Carotenoids and better vision

A diet rich in spinach and other dark green leafy vegetables may help prevent macular degeneration, the leading cause of blindness among people over forty.

The macula is a small dimple in the retina that is responsible for central vision, which is required for writing, sewing, driving, and distinguishing color. Macular degeneration is very common; 65 percent of all sixty-five-year-olds have clinical evidence for this disease. The cause of macular degeneration is unknown, although it is suspected that free radical damage due to long-term exposure to visible light and UV radiation may be responsible. Several animal studies have shown that when deprived of antioxidants, many different species, including primates, our closest relatives in the animal kingdom, are likely to develop retinal degeneration. Studies also show that exposure to bright light also accelerates retinal degeneration in animals. There is no cure or effective treatment for macular degeneration, but recently, researchers have offered one ray of hope. It appears as if two carotenoids, lutein and zeaxanthin, may help to prevent this disease.

According to a study conducted at Harvard Medical School under the direction of Dr. Johanna M. Seddon, people who ate a diet rich in two dark green leafy vegetables, spinach and collard greens, had a substantially reduced risk of developing age-related macular degeneration than those who did not. What is particularly intriguing about this finding is that spinach and collard greens are excellent sources of lutein and zeaxanthin. These are the only two known carotenoids found in very high concentrations in the macula region of the eye.

Researchers have speculated that these two carotenoids may protect the macula against free radical damage. Interestingly, intake of vitamins C and E did not appear to reduce the risk of macular degeneration, although we know that these vitamins may protect against cataracts. Once again, I want to stress that there is no evidence that lutein and zeaxanthin supplements will work as well as foods rich in these carotenoids. Further studies are needed to determine whether supplements will help. My advice is to eat an abundance of fruits and vegetables, especially dark green leafy vegetables.

If you won't eat fruits and vegetables because you don't like them, or are particularly concerned about macular degeneration, you can take a mixed carotenoid supplement that includes a small amount of lutein and zeaxanthin in addition to other carotenoids. We don't know if this will be as effective as obtaining carotenoids through food, but my hunch is that it's better than nothing.

Although taking carotenoids in supplement form is controversial, there is absolutely no controversy regarding the importance of eating an abundance of fruits and vegetables. Food is one of the safest and most effective ways to boost the antioxidant network, and to maximize health and minimize illness. If you are not eating enough fruits and vegetables, or don't know which ones are the best sources of antioxidants, be sure to read chapter 13, An Antioxidant Feast. It will show you how easy it is to incorporate antioxidants into your diet.

11

The Selenium
Surprise

* Selenium is not an antioxidant, but it is an essential component of two important antioxidant enzymes. Selenium also works in synergy with vitamin E.
* Selenium protects against many different forms of cancer, including lung, prostate, and colon cancer.
* People who live in areas where there is little selenium in the soil are at higher risk of dying from stroke and heart disease.
* *RDA:* 50 to 100 micrograms daily.
* *The Packer Plan:* I recommend a supplement of 200 micrograms daily.
* *Sources:* Selenium is not produced by the body and must be obtained through food and water. Food sources of selenium include garlic, onions, wheat germ, red grapes, broccoli, and egg yolks.

Selenium gives credence to the adage, "Good things come in small packages." Although selenium is a trace mineral—we need only a minuscule amount—it offers powerful protection against many different diseases and is an important supporting player in the antioxidant defense network.

Although selenium is beneficial in small amounts, in high doses it can be toxic. The doses that I recommend, however, are well within the safe and beneficial range.

Selenium was discovered in 1817 but was not identified as important for human and animal health until 1957. It wasn't until the past two decades, however, that we began to fully appreciate the important role selenium plays in the antioxidant network.

This mineral never ceases to surprise us. Although selenium is not an antioxidant, it is necessary for the production of several enzymes that affect the antioxidant network. These include glutathione peroxidase, which recycles glutathione and is important for the removal of toxic by-products of lipid peroxidation, and thioredoxin reductase, which recycles vitamin C. Selenium also has a synergistic effect with vitamin E, which means that the two combined are more powerful than either one alone.

The RDA for selenium is 75 micrograms for men and 55 micrograms for women. Many Americans do not consume even this small amount of selenium in their daily diet.

Not consuming enough selenium could be dangerous to your health. Both low consumption of selenium-rich foods and low blood levels of selenium have been strongly associated with an increased risk of heart attack, stroke, and many different types of cancer.

Selenium and your heart

The selenium content in food and water varies from region to region, depending on the selenium content in the soil. Dr. Raymond Shamberger of the Cleveland Clinic, an early proponent of selenium's role in human health, discovered that people who lived in states with the lowest selenium soil content were three times more likely to die of heart disease than those who lived in states that were more selenium-rich. The selenium-deficient states include Connecticut, Illinois, Ohio, Oregon, Massachusetts, Rhode Island, New York, Pennsylvania, Indiana and Delaware, as well as the District of Columbia.

If you live in a selenium-deficient area, you may want to consider moving to Colorado Springs, which has the highest selenium content in its soil and one of the lowest death rates from heart disease in the United States.

The "selenium advantage" is not unique to North America—it holds true throughout the world. One famous Finnish study showed that people who lived in areas with the highest concentration of selenium in the drinking water had significantly lower death rates from heart disease than those who lived in areas with the lowest concentration.

How does selenium protect against heart disease? There are several explanations. First, selenium is necessary for the activity of antioxidant enzymes that can detoxify rancid fat in membranes. There are several enzymes that need selenium and in times of need, these enzymes will hold on to it more tightly.

Second, human platelets contain more selenium than any other tissues, which suggests that the high concentration of selenium in platelets may prevent blood clots.

Now that we know about the workings of the antioxidant network, I believe that selenium's role goes even further. It goes to the very heart of the antioxidant network—vitamin E. Vitamin E is the body's primary fat-soluble antioxidant, which protects lipoproteins against oxidative damage. By adding selenium to the mix, vitamin E can do its job better, which will boost its antioxidant power.

Let me tell you about a fascinating medical mystery that was only recently solved, and everyone was surprised by the ending. In Nianning County, China, residents were particularly vulnerable to Keshan's disease, a rare form of cardiomyopathy that primarily strikes children and women of child-bearing age. It was known that the soil in Nianning is especially low in selenium. Since the residents of Nianning ate primarily food grown in their region, researchers concluded that many were selenium-deficient, and perhaps selenium supplements could have a beneficial effect. In 1974, researchers initiated a double-blind, controlled study in which they gave one group of children selenium supplements, and another group a placebo. Within two years, Keshan's disease had virtually vanished among the group taking the selenium supplements, and the trial was discontinued. From that point on, all children were given selenium supplements, and the incidence of Keshan's disease quickly plummeted.

On the surface, it appeared as if Keshan's disease was simply caused by a nutritional deficiency, and that selenium cured the disease by fortifying the antioxidant defenses of the heart. But in science, as in life, first impressions are often wrong. Further studies performed by Orville Levander of the USDA found that Keshan's disease was actually triggered by a virus that attacked the heart, and that either vitamin E or selenium could protect against the cardiomyopathy caused by this disease.

Scientists have hypothesized that either selenium or vitamin E, or perhaps both, may prevent cardiomyopathy by suppressing the activity of the viral genes that are essential for the virus to spread. In other words, even if a virus attempts to invade the body, if there are plenty of antioxidants on guard, the virus will be less able to reproduce and, therefore, will be stopped in its tracks. This surprise ending shows that when it comes to scientific research, half of the battle is simply knowing what to look for. It also provides further proof of a central theme of *The Antioxidant Miracle:* Antioxidants are not just the body's free radical police.

Selenium and the AIDS connection

As we learn more about antioxidants, it is becoming apparent that they are involved in the progression, if not the onset, of numerous diseases, including AIDS—acquired immune deficiency syndrome. Although linked by a common virus, AIDS is actually a group of diseases that results from the destruction of the immune system. AIDS is caused by the human immunodeficiency virus (HIV), which, although it is slow-acting, is particularly lethal because over time it can knock out T-cells, the main disease-fighting cells of the immune system. As a result, people with HIV are more prone to develop so-called opportunistic infections that attack a weakened body, such as pneumonia and cytomegalovirus, which can cause blindness. When a person with a well-functioning immune system encounters these infections, they are usually able to fight them off. Not so with an HIV-infected person.

AIDS patients have a common link: They are extremely deficient in both glutathione and selenium. Low levels of these two key antioxidants can place AIDS patients under extreme oxidative stress, which will only further weaken their immune function. As you may recall, I have said that low levels of glutathione are a marker for death and disease in people of all ages, and in fact, AIDS patients with the lowest levels of glutathione have the highest mortality rate. Since selenium is essential for the production of glutathione peroxidase, boosting your selenium levels by taking supplements is a good way to protect glutathione.

People infected with HIV need to be especially vigilant about taking supplemental antioxidants, as well as eating an antioxidant-rich diet. In particular, it is important to avoid cigarette smoke, excessive alcohol consumption, and drugs that can further exacerbate oxidative stress.

Selenium: the cancer fighter

Garlic, onion, broccoli, and whole grains are on the National Cancer Institute's list of foods that can reduce your risk of developing cancer. Along with other phytochemicals, these foods are all rich in selenium.

As far back as the 1960s, researchers speculated that low blood levels of selenium may be associated with an increased risk of cancer. Through the years, scientists have built a persuasive case that a selenium-rich diet may protect against cancer. What's even more exciting, recent studies offer compelling evidence that selenium supplements may greatly reduce the risk of many different common cancers.

There are numerous studies that have linked low selenium levels with higher cancer rates. One of the most famous is the so-called Willet study, which was published in the British medical journal *Lancet* in 1983. Headed by Dr. Walter C. Willet of Harvard, this study was conducted at several research centers throughout the United States. In 1973, blood samples were collected from 4,480 men in fourteen regions of the country. At the time the blood was taken, none of the men had any signs of cancer. Over the next five years, 111 men from this group developed cancer. The blood samples of the men who developed cancer were analyzed against a group of 210 healthy men who were similar in age and lifestyle, except that they had not developed cancer. The researchers found that the men with the lowest blood levels of selenium (in the lowest 20 percent) were twice as likely to have developed cancer as those with the highest levels.

The following year, Cornell University researchers compared the blood selenium levels of skin cancer patients to those who did not have cancer. Once again, they found that those with the lowest levels of blood selenium (in the lowest 10 percent) were 5.8 times as likely to have skin cancer as those in the highest group.

The strong correlation between selenium levels and skin cancer led to another study sponsored by the National Cancer Institute at seven dermatology clinics in the United States. In the study, 1,312 patients ranging from ages eighteen to eighty with a history of basal cell or squamous cell skin carcinoma were given either 200 micrograms of selenium daily or a placebo. Patients were followed for about eight years. The study was established to determine whether selenium supplements would prevent a recurrence of skin cancer. Much to the disappointment of the researchers, it did not. In fact, there was virtually no difference in the recurrence of cancer in the selenium-supplemented group versus the placebo-taking group. It appeared as if the study was a dismal failure.

Once again, appearances proved to be deceptive. As researchers analyzed the data, they were astonished by what they found.

The selenium takers had much lower rates of many other kinds of cancers, especially those affecting the lung, prostate, and colon. In fact, the group taking selenium had *half* the death rate from cancer that the placebo takers had. The question remains, why didn't selenium reduce the recurrence of skin cancer? The researchers speculate that selenium's power over cancer may be purely preventive, and that once cancer takes hold, the mineral may not be able to stop it.

Those of us who have devoted our careers to the study of antioxidants understand that antioxidants can be powerful preventive medicine, and that is why so many of us take antioxidant supplements ourselves.

Given what we know about the antioxidant network, it is unlikely that selenium alone is responsible for the reduction in cancer rates, but rather it is yet another example of the close relationship between network antioxidants and their boosters. Selenium is necessary for the production of enzymes needed to make glutathione, which in turn recycles vitamin C, which in turn recharges E. Selenium also synergizes with vitamin E, thereby enhancing its action. Undoubtedly, by bolstering the entire network, selenium gives the body added ammunition to fight against cancer and other diseases.

As we learn more about antioxidants, I have no doubt that we will be in for many more surprises. The network antioxidants and their boosters keep us sharp, strong, and resilient. I have shown why it is critical to maintain the antioxidant advantage, and why losing it can be so devastating to both the body and the mind.

Based on work performed at the Packer Lab, and at other labs like it, I believe that there is a strong body of evidence to confirm the power of the antioxidant network, and more specifically, that a combination of antioxidants will work better than any single antioxidant.

12

Fulfilling the Antioxidant Miracle
Achieving Optimal Health

The antioxidant network:

* Keeps your body youthful

* Bolsters your natural defenses against cancer

* Prevents and even reverses heart disease

* Sharpens your mental edge

Boosting the antioxidant network through diet and supplements can have a profound effect on the length and, more important, the quality of our lives. The key to healthy aging is to fortify the body with the tools it needs to stay healthy. Thanks to our new understanding of the antioxidant network, we can enjoy longer, happier, and more fulfilling lives.

The antioxidant network bolsters the body's natural ability to fight disease and maintain youthful vitality by keeping our cells young, our hearts strong, and our brains functioning at their peak.

In past chapters, I have described the benefits of each of the network antioxidants and booster antioxidants, and I highlighted their unique characteristics.

Now I will show you the full power of the Antioxidant Miracle put together. You will see how the combined antioxidant network can prevent and even reverse the most common health concerns: heart disease, cancer, diminished brain function, and aging.

Preventing heart disease

A strong antioxidant network can provide powerful protection against the number one killer of men and women—heart disease. Heart disease is very much a disease of aging in that it primarily strikes people in middle age and beyond. In fact, one out of two people will eventually die of heart disease. Heart disease is the leading cause of death in men age thirty-nine and older. By age sixty, it is the leading cause of death in women as well.

The first sign of heart disease is a heart attack, yet the foundation for heart disease is laid decades earlier when plaque deposits begin to develop in the arteries delivering blood to the heart. Over time, the plaque grows, and eventually it can block the blood flow leading to the heart.

Lifestyle plays a major role in whether or not we will succumb to heart disease. Smoking, poor diet, and a sedentary and stressful lifestyle are factors that promote heart disease. An antioxidant-rich diet combined with my supplement regimen can help to keep your heart healthy and strong.

In particular, lipoic acid, the vitamin E family and vitamin C, Co Q10, and the flavonoids should make a huge difference in maintaining a healthy heart.

Although all of the network antioxidants are important, studies are beginning to provide proof that vitamin E is the most powerful heart-healthy vitamin. More than forty years ago, my friend and colleague A. L. Tappel discovered that vitamin E prevented lipid peroxidation, which is caused by free radicals and can damage fats and proteins in the body. Today we believe that lipid peroxidation is the underlying cause of heart disease.

If lipid peroxidation is the primary cause of heart disease, and vitamin E can prevent it, then it stands to reason that people who ingest the most vitamin E through food or supplements should have the lowest rates of heart disease. After decades of research, that is precisely the conclusion reached by many different researchers.

THE MORE VITAMIN E, THE LESS HEART DISEASE   In a major cross-cultural study performed in twenty different European populations, scientists found that people who lived in northern Europe were at much greater risk of dying from heart disease than people who lived in the south. The difference was striking: 350 to 400 deaths annually per 100,000 people in the north as opposed to 100 deaths annually per 100,000 people in the south. Why was the mortality from heart disease so high in the north, and so much lower in the south? There are several answers to this question, and they all point to the heart-saving power of vitamin E.

First, researchers found there was a direct correlation between high blood cholesterol levels and death from heart disease: the populations with the highest blood cholesterol levels had the greatest risk of dying from heart disease. This makes sense since high blood cholesterol levels are an indication of high levels of LDL, the "bad cholesterol," which is most vulnerable to peroxidation.

Researchers also found that populations with the highest amount of vitamin E in their blood plasma had the lowest rate of death from heart disease. This finding is a reflection of the healthy diet of southern Europeans—the so-called Mediterranean diet— which includes high amounts of beneficial vitamin E–rich foods, such as olive oil and assorted fruits and green vegetables, as well as other antioxidant-rich foods and beverages.

When researchers compared eight populations with the same average blood cholesterol levels, it was found that those with the highest blood levels of vitamin E had the lowest rate of heart disease. No matter how they played the numbers, vitamin E still emerged as the hero.

The most dramatic study to date attesting to the benefits of vitamin E was performed on patients who had already been diagnosed with one heart attack. The Cambridge Heart Antioxidant Study (known as CHAOS) was a double-blind, placebo-controlled study of 2,002 people with diagnosed heart disease. Patients were given either vitamin E supplements or a placebo. Within 510 days, researchers found that the patients who had been taking vitamin E had an amazing 77 percent fewer heart attacks than those who did not take vitamin E. With such good results, researchers decided to discontinue the study and pre-scribe vitamin E to all of the patients.

The alpha tocopherol portion of the vitamin E family is believed to be the one that protects LDL from oxidation. But that is not the only way that vitamin protects against heart disease. In the chapter on vitamin E, I described a recent study that showed that tocotrienols, a member of the vitamin E family, can literally clean out arteries filled with plaque deposits. In the study, the physician gave tocotrienols or a placebo to patients with carotid stenosis, or a blockage of their carotid artery in the neck. An astonishing 94 percent of the patients receiving tocotrienols improved or stabilized, whereas none of the controls improved, and over half got worse. In all likelihood, tocotrienols can perform the same magic in the arteries delivering blood to the heart.

VITAMIN C AND THE FLAVONOIDS   Vitamin E doesn't do the job alone. Since vitamin C is the network antioxidant that recycles vitamin E, it is also essential for a healthy heart. A major study conducted by James E. Enstrom of the University of California found that people who consumed more than 50 milligrams of vitamin C daily had a signifi-cantly lower risk of death from heart disease than those who did not.

Flavonoids (such as ginkgo and Pycnogenol) are important to the network because they can extend the life of vitamin C, which in turn, boosts levels of vitamin E. These antioxidants also improve circulation, which provides blood and oxygen to the heart muscle. In addition, they are important free radical scavengers.

CO Q10 REVERSES HEART FAILURE   Co Q10 also recycles vitamin E, helping the body to maintain the antioxidant advantage against heart disease. There have been several remarkable studies, notably those performed by Dr. Peter Langsjoen and my friend, the late Dr. Karl Folkers, that showed that Co Q10 was nothing short of miraculous in the treatment of heart failure. That is why I recommend that people who have a family history of heart disease take Co Q10 supplements.

LIPOIC ACID PREVENTS HEART DAMAGE   The role of lipoic acid in preventing heart disease should not be overlooked either. The Packer Lab has demonstrated that lipoic acid can protect the heart against the damaging effects of free radicals. It does not take a great leap of faith to conclude that lipoic acid is having a similar effect on human hearts.

All of the network antioxidants in general, and lipoic acid in particular, can help prevent diabetes, a virtual epidemic in the United States, and a disease that greatly increases the risk of developing heart disease. Diabetics live in a state of oxidative stress, which means that they have too many free radicals and too few antioxidants. That is precisely the scenario that is most likely to breed heart disease.

When it comes to heart disease, the antioxidant network and its boosters work in synergy for our benefit and help to defeat a common disease of aging.

Preventing cancer

One of the most exciting areas of scientific research involves the role of antioxidants in the prevention and treatment of cancer. I believe that strengthening the network antioxidant system, as I recommend in the Packer Plan, will, over time, greatly reduce the risk of many different types of cancers.

At the dawn of the new century, cancer is the second most common cause of death in North America and, if present trends continue, may become the leading cause of death early in the 2000s.

Cancer is not inevitable; in fact, most cancers can be prevented by making simple changes in lifestyle. Abstaining from known carcinogens such as cigarette smoke, eating an abundance of fresh fruits and vegetables, and getting regular exercise can greatly reduce your risk of getting cancer. It is no coincidence that a decade or two after suntans became fashionable, cases of skin cancer began to rise. Nor is it a coincidence that lung cancer has exceeded breast cancer as the number one killer of women. You can track the rise in lung cancer cases with the rise in female smoking after World War II. Cancer may be a complex disease, but the prevention of cancer is not always complex.

Throughout this book, I have described numerous studies that clearly show a dramatic decrease in cancer rates among people who either eat diets rich in antioxidants or, to a lesser extent, take antioxidant supplements. Although there have been numerous studies linking a diet rich in antioxidants with a reduction in cancer, there have been few studies involving antioxidant supplements.

Although antioxidants are not the magic cure for cancer, the evidence is overwhelming that antioxidants play an important role in protecting against cancer. The network antioxidants and their boosters work by bolstering the body's ability to defeat cancer before it can take hold. Unlike drugs that are designed to eradicate disease after the fact, the primary job of antioxidants is to fortify the body's own defense mechanisms against disease.

There are several ways antioxidants can strengthen our resistance to cancer. There are many different forms of cancer, but basically all forms involve the abnormal growth of cells. Whatever the cause, the cancer process begins when a cell mutates and begins to multiply wildly. If allowed to grow, these cancerous cells invade healthy cells, robbing them of their nutrients. In a sense, cancer kills us by starvation.

Free radical damage to DNA, the genetic material within every cell, can cause a cell to mutate and begin to divide erratically. On the most basic level, antioxidants protect the DNA in genes from free radical attack. A strong antioxidant defense system can stop free radicals before they can attack DNA.

ANTIOXIDANTS BOOST THE IMMUNE SYSTEM   Antioxidants can also enhance the ability of the immune system to weed out cancer cells. For example, high intakes of vitamins C and E are associated with lower rates of many different types of cancers. I believe that these antioxidants may be effective because they are boosting immune function. Our immune system not only protects us against infectious diseases, but one of its primary functions is to maintain a lookout for cancerous cells and to destroy them before they do harm. If the immune system is vigorous, it should be able to take out cancer cells before they cause damage. However, as we age and levels of network antioxidants such as glutathione and Co Q10 decline, there is a marked drop in immune function. There is also a dramatic increase in the risk of developing cancer. Antioxidant supplementation—especially vitamin E—has been shown to reinvigorate immune function in both older animals and people. Undoubtedly, this added boost to immune function means better protection against cancer.

ANTIOXIDANTS REGULATE GENES   But antioxidants have an even more profound impact in helping to stave off cancer. As noted earlier, we have discovered that antioxidants can turn on and off genes that regulate cell growth. A cell has no mind of its own; it is controlled by genes that tell it precisely what to do and when to do it. In order for genes to send messages to cells, they must be activated or turned on. Free radicals and carcinogens can turn on bad genes that tell cells to mutate. Antioxidants can shut down these bad genes. Eventually, I foresee a new generation of cancer treatments that will harness the power of antioxidants to control cancer at its most fundamental level.

Antioxidants can have a profound effect on people who may be at risk of developing cancer because of their family history. It is commonly believed that a gene for a particular form of cancer is passed down from parent to child. There are genes that are specific to certain types of cancer—for example, there is a gene for colon cancer and other genes for breast cancer. In most cases, however, you do not inherit a gene for a specific type of cancer, but rather you inherit a weakness in the genes that control the body's natural enzyme detoxification system. This means that over time, your body will lose its ability to fight against carcinogens, leaving you vulnerable to many different types of cancer.

ANTIOXIDANTS BOLSTER THE DETOXIFICATION SYSTEM Almost half of Americans have less than optimal combinations of two key enzyme detoxification systems—the glutathione and the cytochrome P450 family. As we age, these natural protective systems become exhausted by overload. The good news is that the antioxidant network and, in particular, lipoic acid, play two important protective roles. First, they boost glutathione levels, compensating for inherited weaknesses. Second, they turn on the process called apoptosis in which bad cells self-destruct before they can infect healthy cells.

Population studies examining diet and cancer have led to some remarkable discoveries. From these studies, we now know that lycopene, an antioxidant found in tomatoes, may provide powerful protection against prostate cancer. We have learned that people who drink green tea, a good source of flavonoids, have markedly lower levels of cancer than those who don't. We also know that cruciferous vegetables (such as broccoli and kale) have special antioxidants that can inhibit the growth of tumors. In chapter 13, I expand further on the cancer-fighting potential of antioxidants in food.

Recently, there has been some intriguing information on the use of single antioxidants to treat cancer:

* A form of vitamin E, tocotrienols, has been shown to inhibit the growth of breast cancer cells in the test tube.

* According to a new study reported in the *Journal of the National Cancer Institute,* men who took at least 50 milligrams of vitamin E daily were 32 percent less likely to develop prostate cancer and 42 percent less likely to die from it.

* In another major study conducted in cooperation with the National Cancer Institute, selenium takers had much lower rates of cancer, especially those affecting the lung, prostate, and colon.

* Researchers have reported remarkable success in using Co Q10 along with other therapies as a treatment for advanced breast cancer.

Clearly, antioxidants are an integral part of the body's natural system of checks and balances to control the initiation and spread of cancer. Keeping the antioxidant network strong through food and supplements and reducing exposure to carcinogens can result in a significant decline in the cases of new cancers in the twenty-first century.

Keeping your brain young

Even before many of us notice our first gray hair or our first wrinkle, we may experience one of the earliest signs of aging: the loss of short-term memory. By age forty, many people begin to find that they are not as sharp as they used to be in remembering names, or where they put the car keys. In reality, although it can be annoying, this type of memory loss is not a sign of a more serious problem such as Alzheimer's disease. Nor does it mean that you are not as smart as you used to be. These symptoms of short-term memory loss are merely a sign of wear and tear on the brain. Keeping your network antioxidants at optimal levels can help reduce and perhaps even reverse these symptoms. There is also good evidence that they may prevent these minor problems from developing into more serious age-related brain disorders.

Your brain is particularly vulnerable to free radical damage for two reasons. First, it is a hotbed of activity; it never stops working. Brain cells need a constant flow of blood and oxygen to produce energy, which increases the production of free radicals. Second, the brain is composed of 50 percent fat, which makes it vulnerable to lipid peroxidation. At the same time as we age, there is a decline in hormones and other chemicals in the brain that regulate our memory, learning, and ability to reason.

Replenishing antioxidants through foods and supplements that I recommend in the Packer Plan will help your brain regain its antioxidant advantage and will keep your mental edge sharp.

Several studies have already shown that antioxidants can make a real difference in brain function.

Ginkgo Biloba

Of all the network antioxidants and their boosters, ginkgo biloba, a flavonoid, has become best known as the antioxidant for your brain. In Europe, ginkgo is commonly prescribed for mental problems that are often caused by poor circulation to the brain, such as difficulty concentrating, poor memory, depression, and anxiety. In the United States, ginkgo biloba is one of the top-selling herbs.

Ginkgo works by helping to control nitric oxide, an important free radical. Nitric oxide modulates communication among brain cells and is instrumental in helping us concentrate, learn new information, and maintain memories. But if not tightly controlled, nitric oxide can wreak havoc on brain cells. There have been numerous European studies performed on ginkgo, and many have reported positive effects in memory and acuity. Recently, ginkgo extract was tested on patients suffering from dementia (caused by either stroke or Alzheimer's disease) with somewhat positive results.

Vitamin E

Animal and test tube studies have strongly suggested that vitamin E may play a role in preventing Alzheimer's disease by protecting brain cells against free radical attack. Recently, vitamin E has also been found to help slow down the progression of mental decline in patients with Alzheimer's disease. Although we don't know the cause of Alzheimer's, it is believed that free radicals are involved in the progression, if not the onset, of Alzheimer's disease as well as other degenerative brain diseases. The brain tissue of Alzheimer's patients typically has higher levels of lipid peroxidation, a sign of oxidative damage, than disease-free people of the same age. We have performed numerous experiments in my laboratory that demonstrate that vitamin E (along with Coenzyme Q10, the other fat-soluble antioxidant) can reduce lipid peroxidation in the brain.

Many researchers suspect that free radical damage to neurons may inhibit the ability of nerve cells to produce adequate levels of neurotransmitters and other chemicals in the brain that organize thought processes and help brain cells communicate. As we get older, there is a natural decline in the production of neurotransmitters, which is a factor in normal brain aging. However, this decline may be greatly accelerated in the brains of Alzheimer's patients. It is my hope that taking antioxidants early in life will prevent some of the brain damage that occurs later in life.

Lipoic Acid

Although it is not widely known, I believe that lipoic acid one day soon may supplant ginkgo biloba and vitamin E as the antioxidant for the brain. In my laboratory, we have had some spectacular results using lipoic acid on animals who have suffered from stroke, and we have shown that lipoic acid can completely prevent stroke-related brain damage, which is primarily caused by free radicals. If lipoic acid can prevent brain injury during an acute free radical attack, such as that experienced during a stroke, then I believe over time it will protect the brain from the free radical attack normally experienced every day.

Co Q10

Recently, I learned of a study that strongly suggested that Co Q10, which boosts vitamin E levels in the network, could slow down or even reverse some of the common age-related brain disorders. Under the direction of Flint Beal, M.D., researchers at Massachusetts General Hospital gave laboratory mice a toxic drug called malonate, which kills brain cells. These mice were also specially bred to develop amyotrophic lateral sclerosis (ALS). When given the brain poison malonate, ALS mice typically develop big lesions in their brains that rapidly destroy brain tissue, leading to rapid death. However, when Dr. Beal administered Co Q10 along with the malonate, the mice showed substantially less brain damage and lived an average of eight days longer. This study proved that Co Q10 was able to provide protection for brain cells under the most trying conditions of oxidative stress. To me this suggests that Co Q10 should also help control free radical attack under more normal, less severe conditions in healthy older brains.

Slowing down the aging process

Recently, I was at a dinner party where I struck up a conversation with a man who asked me about my work. When I told him about the Packer Lab, the antioxidant network, and how I believed that antioxidants might ultimately extend life, his response surprised me. Instead of being excited at the prospect of living longer, he was negative. He raised an important, common question: Why extend life if we are condemned to spend those last years in sickness and disability? He went on to describe how Alzheimer's disease had eroded his father's mental function until he was unable to perform even the most menial of tasks. Drained emotionally and financially by trying to care for his father at home, the son was eventually forced to place his father in a nursing home.

"I'd rather die young than have to live that way," he said grimly.

Frankly, I couldn't agree more. There is no point to adding years to our lives if those years are devoid of any quality of life. But as I see it, it doesn't have to be that way. Old age need not be synonymous with debility and illness.

It is now possible to live a long, high-quality life in a strong, vigorous body—as the ancient Greeks used to say, "To die as *young* as possible as *old* as possible." That is why I find it is impossible to talk about aging without talking about health because the two are so inextricably linked. It is not aging that we should fear; the real enemy is the *disease* of aging.

At any age, disease can accelerate the aging process. Very often, a forty-year-old who is chronically ill will not feel—or look—as youthful as a healthy, vital sixty- or seventy-year-old.

The strategic use of network antioxidants, as I suggest in the Packer Plan, can halt and even reverse many of the problems that have become associated with aging.

Today, although people are living longer than ever before, there is a maximum human life span of about 120, which only a very few people actually achieve. Most people die decades earlier, usually of disease.

Longevity is a complicated issue that is based on both genetics and environment. Clearly, some of us are born more genetically blessed than others. We do inherit a predisposition to develop diseases such as cancer or heart disease, the two leading killers in the Western world. But genetics is not the only factor in determining health; in fact, it plays a relatively minor role. Most of the diseases that cut life short are not caused by bad genes, but by bad habits and a bad environment.

Some 75 to 80 percent of all human cancers are caused by smoking, exposure to pollutants, and especially poor diet. There is equally strong evidence that heart disease is caused by smoking and poor diet. What antioxidants may do (combined with a healthy lifestyle) is increase the odds of living out your life without succumbing to a disease that will destroy the quality of your life and shorten it.

There is also compelling evidence that antioxidants can have a real impact on the mysterious force we call "the aging process." Although there are several theories about why we age, there are no solid answers. Whether there is an "aging clock" in our brains that controls why and how we age, or whether each cell is programmed to self-destruct at a given time, is the subject of much debate.

There is no debate, however, that free radicals are involved in triggering or accelerating the aging process, and that antioxidants can slow down the forces that age us. The free radical theory of aging first proposed by my friend and colleague Denham Harman blames aging on cumulative damage to cells and tissues inflicted over many decades by exposure to free radicals. There is much evidence to prove that he is right.

The free radical theory of aging could just have easily been called the antioxidant theory of longevity. In nature, there is a direct link between high levels of antioxidants and life span.

The protective effect of antioxidants is particularly striking if you correlate the average life spans of different mammalian species with their level of antioxidants. In every case, the species with the greatest amount of vitamin E or the strongest antioxidant defense systems are the longest lived. Humans and elephants top the list in both antioxidant activity and life span, while mice and other rodents with low levels of antioxidants are the shortest lived.

In studies of human cells, we have solid evidence that antioxidants can prevent aging on the cellular level, where the aging process begins. Numerous studies conducted in my lab and others have shown that antioxidants can prevent many of the telltale cellular signs of aging. Since groups of cells form tissues, groups of tissues form organs, and groups of organs are what run our bodies, it makes sense that once our cells begin to age, our bodies simply cannot function well or efficiently.

CELLS LIVE LONGER   Studies have shown that several different antioxidants can extend the life of human cells, primarily by protecting them against free radical damage. As you may recall, I described an experiment performed earlier in my laboratory in which we doubled the life span of human cells simply by adding vitamin E to their culture. What this and similar experiments prove is that exposure to free radicals can shorten life, and that by controlling free radicals, antioxidants can extend life. It's as simple as that.

ANTIOXIDANTS PREVENT TELLTALE SIGNS OF CELLULAR AGING
Antioxidants can prevent one of the telltale signs of cellular aging—the accumulation of an age pigment called lipofuscin in all the specialized cells of the body, but especially in the brain and heart. Lipofuscin is a direct result of lipid peroxidation, or the oxidation of proteins and lipids. Over time, lipofuscin can destroy these organs, fast-forwarding the aging process. In the test tube—and we believe in the body—antioxidants can slow down the formation of lipofuscin dramatically, keeping the cells youthful for a longer period of time.

ANTIOXIDANTS CONTROL AGE   Antioxidants can also prevent another well-known age accelerator—the formation of AGE (advanced glycation end products), which are created by a process called glycation that damages protein. Glycation occurs when glucose reacts with proteins resulting in cross-linking of proteins as well as the formation of free radicals. A high number of these proteins can lead to outer signs of premature aging, such as wrinkles and brown spots on the skin, and can cause even more destruction inside the body. Heart disease, cataracts, arthritis, and even Alzheimer's disease have been associated with the cross-linking of proteins. The universal antioxidant lipoic acid as well as other antioxidants can control the formation of AGE, which in the long run can have a profound effect on every organ system within the body.

I believe that there is no better way to extend life than to keep your antioxidant defense network strong, so that it can control the forces that advance the aging process, including heart disease.

I have been taking antioxidants for several decades, and although I have reached the age at which many Americans retire from their careers, I personally have not experienced the mental slowdown that has become associated with midlife and beyond. In fact, some of my most creative work in terms of unraveling the mysteries of the antioxidant network were performed when I was in my sixties. I still write books, lecture, attend international conferences, do research, run a laboratory, and have enough stamina left over to go sailing on the weekends. I can say the same for many of my fellow antioxidant researchers. Although we are in the seventh and eighth decades, we are still making major contributions to our fields of expertise. I do not consider any of us to be extraordinary; rather we are simply ordinary people who are experiencing the extraordinary benefits of the antioxidant network.

By now, I hope you want to begin the Packer Plan, a comprehensive antioxidant regimen based on the antioxidant network. In Part Four, The Packer Plan: Making the Antioxidant Miracle Work for You, I will tell you everything you need to know to begin the Packer Plan, and to keep your antioxidant defense system in peak condition.

The Packer Plan

Making the Antioxidant Miracle Work for You

13

An Antioxidant Feast: Food Is Powerful Medicine
From Apples to Winter Squash

To keep our antioxidant network strong and effective, we must constantly replenish the antioxidants we lose every second of every day as we carry on our normal activities. What we eat can make a huge difference in our ability to maintain the antioxidant advantage, and to keep our bodies and minds functioning at optimal levels.

The Packer Plan: seven to ten servings of antioxidant-rich fruits and vegetables a day

Why would a serious scientist like me be interested in food? I have to admit, at one time I may have bristled at the notion that something as fundamental as diet could be even more important than the miracles we scientists produce in our laboratories. Today, I know better.

Ironically, despite all of the spectacular, high-tech medical breakthroughs of the twentieth century, Americans are still two to four times more likely to die of lifestyle-related diseases such as heart disease, cancer, stroke, and diabetes than citizens of poor nations. Why? The answers often lie with what we are putting on our plates.

Until recently, modern medicine has ignored the link between diet and disease. Rather, scientists focused on finding the magic bullets that would wipe disease off the planet. There is no doubt that these modern marvels have vastly improved our health, but they may have given the false impression that no matter how serious the disease, the cure could be found in a well-equipped laboratory. The emphasis on high-tech solutions for common health problems diminished the role of lifestyle in maintaining health. By the end of World War II, people who were concerned about nutrition and health were considered to be food faddists at best or health nuts at worst. Fast-food restaurants offering highly processed, high-fat fare were the rage. Hamburgers, chicken nuggets, and french fries were in; fresh fruits and vegetables were out. Diet was considered so unimportant that few medical schools even offered courses in nutrition.

Although doctors offered lip service to eating a well-balanced diet, few understood what that actually meant. In fact, back in those days, doctors were as likely to engage in unhealthy habits such as smoking cigarettes as their patients.

At the same time, despite our superior medical knowledge, heart disease and cancer were becoming epidemic in the United States and Western Europe, and a handful of innovative researchers began to wonder why. What was particularly striking was that this wasn't the case in other parts of the world. Numerous studies revealed that people who lived in less affluent countries where the diet was rich in whole grains and unprocessed fruits and vegetables had markedly lower rates of cancer and heart disease than in the wealthier, more "advanced" nations.

At first, many mainstream scientists dismissed these findings as pure coincidence or that some populations may be genetically prone to develop different diseases. But when more thoughtful scientists began to take a closer look at these studies, they found that certain foods appeared to be protective against disease. There was no denying that people who ate an abundance of plant foods were healthier and lived longer than people who ate the traditional Western diet.

For the first time, serious scientists began to study these plant foods using the same state-of-the-art techniques that had been previously used only for the most cutting-edge research. In laboratories around the world, scientists began to isolate particular chemicals in fruits, vegetables, and commonly used spices (like garlic and turmeric). These scientists discovered that foods contained a wide array of protective compounds called phytochemicals, many of which were antioxidants.

There are literally hundreds of phytochemicals, many offering unique benefits. For example, cruciferous vegetables such as broccoli have special chemicals that stimulate the production of anticancer compounds in the body. Soybeans are rich in isoflavones, hormonelike compounds that fight cancer. Citrus fruits contain a cancer-fighting oil in their skin. The more that was revealed about fruits and vegetables, the more apparent it became that food was powerful medicine. From this research, we have learned several important lessons:

* First and foremost, there is no substitute for a healthy, well-balanced diet. Supplements can help enhance the health benefits of food, but they cannot do the job alone.

* Many of the important phytochemicals are in the pigments of plants. For example, dark-green leafy vegetables have different phytochemicals from those in yellow and orange vegetables. Therefore, it is important to eat an assortment of brightly colored fruits and vegetables daily to ensure that you are getting a full range of phytochemicals.

* Fresh whole fruits and vegetables are your best option. Although juice has vitamins and minerals, only the whole fruit or vegetable contains fiber. Ideally, you should also eat the skin of the fruit or vegetable since it is a wonderful source of nutrients. Many people, however, are concerned about pesticides, waxes, and other preservatives used on produce to retain color and freshness. You can avoid pesticides and other chemicals by buying organic fruits and vegetables from reputable stores. Be sure to scrub your produce thoroughly before eating it.

* There is no magic bullet—there are so many different phytochemicals in just one vegetable or fruit, it is impossible to say which is the one that is most beneficial. In fact, it is possible that different phytochemicals work together to achieve their effects.

* Limit fat consumption to around 30 percent of your daily calories. Raw, unhydrogenated oils, such as canola oil, olive oil,

flaxseed oil, and peanut oil are the healthiest. Solid fats, such as stick margarine and butter, should be avoided because they promote the formation of disease-promoting fats.

Despite the explosion of information on the benefits of food, few Americans eat the five servings of fruits and vegetables daily recommended by the National Cancer Institute and the American Heart Association. In fact, many don't even eat one serving.

Instead, we are filling our plates with high-fat, high-calorie foods that have resulted in an epidemic of obesity and the diseases that are associated with this condition. In fact, today a record 35 percent of all Americans are considered to be dangerously overweight. Filling our plates with the right food will, over time, eliminate obesity and dramatically reduce the incidence of self-inflicted diseases associated with poor diet.

As part of the Packer Plan, I urge people to make a conscientious effort to eat a wide variety of antioxidant-rich fruits and vegetables daily. I understand that not everyone likes every food. Therefore, I have listed a wide variety of different antioxidant foods for you to choose from.

In most cases, fresh fruits and vegetables are the best sources of vitamins, minerals, and other phytochemicals. There is one important exception, however: vitamin C. Vitamin C is somewhat fragile and can be destroyed in shipping and food handling. Freeze-dried products, such as orange, grapefruit, and cranberry juice, may actually have a higher vitamin C content than the fresh fruit.

Here are some suggestions of fresh fruits and vegetables that are excellent sources of important antioxidants. To keep your antioxidant network at the strongest level, try to eat seven to ten portions of these foods daily.

Eating should not be a chore and I don't want you to worry about portion size. However, keep in mind that *1 medium-size fruit* or *½ cup of cooked or raw vegetables* is usually considered 1 portion.

Apples
Lower cholesterol
Protect against cancer
The powerful combination of flavonoids that enhance the activity of vitamin C in the antioxidant network and fiber may be why "an apple a day keeps the doctor away."

Starting in 1965, researchers at Finland's Public Health Institute in Helsinki followed the dietary habits of 9,959 cancer-free men and women between the ages of fifteen and ninety-nine. In 1991, out of this group, 997 cases of cancer had been diagnosed, 151 of which were lung cancer. When researchers contrasted the diets of those who developed cancer with those who did not, they found that people who regularly ate foods rich in flavonoids were 20 percent less likely to develop cancer than those who did not. Moreover, the flavonoid fans were at a 46 percent lower risk of developing lung cancer. In particular, apples were found to be a highly protective food. Onions were a close second. Researchers speculated that quercetin, a flavonoid that is abundant in both apples and onions, may be the secret ingredient in these foods that fights cancer.

Apples may not only be cancer fighters, but they may also protect against heart disease. Apples are rich in pectin, a type of soluble fiber that has been shown to lower blood cholesterol levels.

Berries
Good for vision
Contain cancer-fighting compounds

Berries, especially blueberries, bilberries (a relative of the American blueberry), and strawberries, are not only good-tasting but are wonderful sources of natural phytochemicals.

Blueberries contain blue pigments called *anthocyanin*, which in test tube studies have been shown to be potent antioxidants. In one study conducted at the USDA, rats fed a few blueberries daily showed fewer signs of mental or physical aging than those that did not eat blueberries. Although the researchers were not sure why blueberries appeared to slow down aging, it could be caused by the antioxidant content. Blueberries, like apples, are also an excellent source of pectin, which can lower blood cholesterol levels.

Bilberry, another rich source of anthocyanin, is a traditional remedy for preserving night vision. Legend has it that during World War II, British pilots would eat bilberry jam before night missions to improve their vision. Anthocyanin may help protect small blood vessels from free radical damage, thereby helping to improve the microcirculation to the eye.

Eating strawberries may protect you from cancer. Strawberries contain a polyphenolic compound called *ellagic acid,* a natural antioxidant that may block the destructive effects of free radicals. Other fruits such as grapes and cherries contain ellagic acid (and so do walnuts). In an intriguing Japanese study, one group of laboratory rats were fed a variety of polyphenolic compounds, while another group was given only ellagic acid. Both groups of rats were then exposed to a potent carcinogen that can induce tongue cancer. The rats given a variety of polyphenolic compounds had a much lower rate of cancer than control rats not given polyphenols. However, quite remarkably, none of the rats fed ellagic acid went on to develop cancer. Not only rats, but humans may be protected from cancer by strawberries.

In a famous study that I describe in greater detail when I discuss tomatoes, Harvard Medical School researchers reported that four foods appeared to be protective against prostate cancer. Since three of the four foods were tomato-based (such as pizza and tomato sauce), both the researchers and the press completely ignored the fourth, non-tomato-based food. The finding that was not widely reported was that men who ate the most strawberries were at the lowest risk of developing prostate cancer.

Recently, scientists at the Ohio State University College of Medicine in Columbus found that black raspberries substantially reduce the cancer risk in rats fed a carcinogen known to induce esophageal cancer.

Studies such as these suggest that berries may be a powerful disease-fighting food. It's important to note, however, that berries contain many different substances, such as fiber, vitamin C, and flavonoids, which have also been proven to be protective against cancer and other diseases related to aging. In addition, berries may contain other compounds that have yet to be discovered. Eat them by the handful!

Carrots
Protect against heart attack and stroke
Contain cancer-fighting compounds

Carrots are a member of the Umbelliferae family (along with celery and parsnips), which has been investigated by the National Cancer Institute for its potential cancer-fighting ability. Cooked carrots contain the highest amounts of the carotenoid alpha carotene of nearly any fruit or vegetable (with the exception of pumpkin). Alpha carotene has been shown to be a potent cancer fighter; in fact, it can suppress the growth of cancerous tumors in animals far better than beta carotene.

Women take note: Carrots can also help protect against stroke. According to the Harvard study of the food consumed by more than 87,000 female nurses, those who had five or more servings a week of carrots were 68 percent less likely to suffer a stroke than those who ate only one serving a month.

Carrots are also rich in beta carotene, which, according to numerous population studies, when consumed in food may reduce the risk of both cancer and cardiovascular disease. Beta carotene is one of the few carotenoids with provitamin A activity; that is, it may be converted in the body to vitamin A as the body needs it.

Even though I am obviously a champion of antioxidants, I am quick to concede that the beneficial effects of carrots do not solely arise from their carotenoids. Carrots are also a wonderful source of calcium pectate, a type of soluble fiber shown to reduce blood cholesterol levels. According to USDA researchers, eating two carrots a day may reduce cholesterol levels in some people by 10 to 20 percent. And those little carrots, prepeeled, washed, and ready-to-eat are a great snack. They are low-calorie, low-fat, and high in fiber.

Citrus Fruits
Protect against many different forms of cancer
A good source of flavonoids, which boost vitamin C
Citrus fruits, including grapefruit, oranges, lemons, limes, tangelos, and tangerines, have been acknowledged by the National Cancer Institute as strong cancer fighters. Well known for being good sources of vitamin C, citrus fruits also contain numerous phytochemicals.

All citrus fruits contain antioxidant flavonoids that enhance vitamin C's action in the antioxidant network.

Pink grapefruit is an excellent source of the carotenoid lycopene, which may protect against prostate cancer in men and cervical cancer in women. (For more information on lycopene, see the entry on tomatoes.)

But perhaps the most important part of the fruit is the one that we routinely discard—the peel. The peels of oranges and lemons contain D-limonene, a citrus oil that in animal studies has been shown to inhibit the growth of breast cancer cells. Limonene belongs to a family of compounds known as *monoterpenes*, which can also reduce cholesterol levels. So, instead of throwing out the peel, grate it into baked goods, or mix it into yogurt or in a fruit salad. To reduce exposure to bacteria from handling and pesticides, be sure to rinse the skin of the fruit well and to scrub it with a vegetable brush before using it in food.

Cruciferous Vegetables
Contain cancer-fighting indoles
May protect against macular degeneration

Cruciferous vegetables, including broccoli, cauliflower, brussels sprouts, cabbage, and kale, have been the subject of intense scientific scrutiny in recent years. These vegetables contain many wonderful phytochemicals, including *sulforaphane* and flavonoids called indole-3-carbinol (indoles), which appear to be powerful cancer fighters.

The first clue that indoles may prevent cancer came from population studies showing that people who consumed large amounts of cruciferous vegetables had a significantly reduced risk of developing certain types of cancers. Intrigued by this finding, researchers at Rockefeller University found that indoles inactivate harmful estrogens that can promote the growth of tumors in estrogen-sensitive cells, particularly in breast cells. Indoles appear to alter the biological pathway that converts estrogen in the body to more harmful forms that stimulate tumor growth. Indoles are being studied as potential chemotherapy drugs. Here is a prime example of how substances with antioxidant activity do much more than simply control free radicals, and how the more we understand their function, the better we can harness their disease-fighting power.

Cruciferous vegetables also contain other potential anticancer compounds such as sulforaphane, and indoles, which stimulate the body to produce cancer-fighting enzymes.

I recommend eating a variety of cruciferous vegetables since each offers a slightly different blend of phytochemicals. For example, kale is an excellent source of the carotenoids lutein and zeaxanthin, which may be protective against macular degeneration. Broccoli contains more sulforaphane than other cruciferous vegetables, as well as antioxidant boosters selenium and beta carotene. All cruciferous vegetables contain fiber, which also reduces cancer risk.

About 25 percent of the population has an inherited aversion to the bitter flavor of cruciferous vegetables. If these veggies taste too much like medicine for your liking, try adding a pinch of salt, which makes cruciferous vegetables taste sweeter.

The nutritional value of cruciferous vegetables is best preserved when they are eaten raw or lightly steamed. Do not boil these vegetables because it will deplete them of indoles. Microwaving them (without added water) just until bright green will help to preserve their antioxidants.

Dried Fruit
Contains cancer-fighting carotenoids

If you have a sweet tooth, dried fruit is a wonderful way to satisfy both your craving for dessert and your body's need for antioxidants. Both dried apricots and peaches are a terrific source of the carotenoid beta carotene. Dried peaches also contain some *cryptoxanthin,* a carotenoid that is being studied for its potential anticancer activity. In addition, these fruits are also a good source of potassium. *Caution:* Sulfites are sometimes added to fruit during the drying process to maintain color. If you are allergic to sulfites, avoid dried fruit or buy fruit processed without sulfites. Diabetics should beware that dried fruit is high in sugar.

Garlic and Onions
Lower cholesterol
Contains cancer-fighting phytochemicals

Garlic and onions belong to the Allium family, which also include leeks and chives. Long before the dawn of modern science, physicians recognized the powerful healing properties of allium vegetables, especially garlic and onions.

Although we use garlic primarily as a flavoring for food, at one time it was considered strong medicine. Hippocrates was reported to have used garlic fumes to treat ovarian cancer. First-century physician Dioscorides wrote that garlic "clears the arteries and opens the mouths of veins." In the Middle Ages, monks chewed on garlic cloves to protect themselves against the plague. Modern scientists have confirmed that garlic is a veritable pharmacy of healing compounds. It is rich in selenium, which provides the building blocks for several enzymes that affect the antioxidant network, including glutathione peroxidase. Garlic is also a heart-healthy herb. Garlic also contains *ajoene,* a compound that prevents blood clots.

In addition, garlic is a rich source of sulphur compounds, which have natural antibiotic and antifungal properties. During World War II, garlic was dubbed Russian penicillin because it was used by the Russian army to fight infection on the battlefield.

As Hippocrates apparently knew, and as modern-day scientists are beginning to discover, garlic may be a potent cancer fighter. Various compounds in garlic can inhibit the growth of cancerous tumors in test tube and animal studies. Recently, German researchers reported that garlic extract prevents breaks in DNA strands that are caused by free radicals, which lead to cancerous changes in cells.

Garlic may also help to thwart the growth of existing cancers. When researchers at Memorial Sloan-Kettering Cancer Research Center exposed prostate cancer cells in culture dishes to a sulphur compound found in aged garlic, S-allylmercaptocysteine, it significantly slowed down their growth. In particular, researchers found that garlic had a positive effect on male hormones. Prostate cancer cells are especially sensitive to a potent metabolite of the male hormone testosterone, dihydrotestosterone, which can stimulate the growth of prostate tumors. But when exposed to S-allylmercaptocysteine, the prostate cancer cells broke down testosterone two to four times faster than normal and did not produce the potentially dangerous DHT. I'm not suggesting that garlic is a cure for cancer, but it certainly can't hurt to add some cooked garlic to your diet.

Onion, a cousin to garlic, is another disease-fighting food. Onion attracted the attention of modern scientists after the *Journal of the National Cancer Institute* published the results of a Chinese study in 1989 reporting that people who ate the highest amounts of onions and other allium vegetables had the lowest rates of stomach cancer. In the study, researchers compared the eating habits of 564 patients with stomach cancer to 1,131 healthy people. They were astonished to find that the primary difference between the two groups was that the cancer-free group ate significantly more allium vegetables.

Onion contains many cancer-fighting compounds. In particular, it is a rich source of the flavonoid *quercetin*, an antioxidant that has been shown in test tube studies to block the action of a variety of natural or synthetic initiators and promoters of cancer cell development. Quercetin is also important as a natural anti-inflammatory and has antibacterial, antifungal, and antiviral activity.

Onion is also an excellent source of selenium, a mineral that has been shown to reduce the risk of many different types of cancer as well as stroke.

Greens
Good for vision
Potent cancer fighter
No phytochemical feast is complete without a serving or two of fresh greens. I'm not talking about the anemic-looking whitish iceberg lettuce that passes for greens; I'm talking about the *real thing*, dark-green leafy vegetables. In North America, we use greens for little more than garnishes to decorate a plate. This is unfortunate, since many greens are loaded with important vitamins (like C and E), minerals (like calcium), and other disease-fighting antioxidants. For example, beet greens, watercress, collard greens, mustard greens, and Swiss chard (all cruciferous vegetables) are excellent sources of the carotenoids lutein and zeaxanthin, which may protect against macular degeneration, and good sources of beta carotene, which may protect against cancer. All greens contain antioxidant flavonoids and mono-terpenes, which can lower cholesterol, and probably a lot of other important compounds we haven't yet identified. Greens are also low in calories and high in fiber. To get the full benefit, eat a mixture of greens lightly steamed. You can also steam greens in a microwave—it will help preserve the phytochemical content.

Red Grapes and Wine
Protect against heart disease
Reduce the risk of stroke
"To your health" is a universal toast that has been translated into virtu-ally every language and has been passed down from countless genera-tions. Wine has been used as both a popular beverage and a medicine for more than 6,000 years. The planting of vineyards was mentioned in Genesis, making grapes the first known crop to be planted by human beings in recorded history.

Scientists began taking a serious look at wine when study after study revealed that moderate wine drinkers not only lived longer than tee-totalers but had a lower incidence of heart disease and even some forms of cancer. Some of you have heard of the French paradox—that is, even though the French eat a diet that is relatively high in fat, and often smoke, they have one of the lowest rates of heart disease in the world. Researchers have theorized that the French may owe their good health to antioxidant compounds found in red wine, and to a lesser extent in red grape juice. The red wine effect appears to be strongest among smokers. Chablis drinkers take note: white wine pales in comparison in terms of health benefits.

Both red wine and red grape juice may protect against heart disease in several ways. First, both of these beverages are an excellent source of phenolic compounds, including catechin, epicatechin, and gallic acid. Although red wine is a better source of phenolic compounds, they are also present in red grape juice. Phenolic compounds have been shown to prevent the formation of blood clots, which are a major cause of both heart attack and stroke in humans.

Second, phenolic compounds also help to modulate the effects of nitric oxide, an important free radical produced by the body. By controlling the muscular tone of blood vessels, nitric oxide regulates circulation and normalizes blood flow, but excessive amounts of nitric oxide can be harmful.

Third, and perhaps most important, phenolic compounds are antioxidants that can prevent the oxidation of LDL cholesterol, which can lead to atherosclerosis and ultimately to a heart attack. Red wine does not lower cholesterol levels, but it does prevent LDL from turning rancid, which can lead to the formation of plaque deposits in arteries.

Wine drinkers are not only less likely to get heart disease, but they appear to be less likely to get macular degeneration, a leading cause of blindness among people over sixty-five. According to an article published in the *Journal of the American Geriatrics Society,* people who drank wine were 20 percent less likely to develop macular degeneration than people who did not drink wine.

Recently, colleagues at the University of California at Davis have investigated whether the phenolic compounds in red wine can help prevent cancer. In animal studies, they have found that when given phenolic compounds from wine, mice bred to develop tumors showed a significant delay in the onset of tumors compared to untreated mice.

There is a second paradox when it comes to wine. Some studies have suggested that women who drink any amount of wine are at a slightly increased risk of developing breast cancer. This may happen because the alcohol in wine boosts estrogen levels, which can stimulate the growth of existing hormone-sensitive tumors. On the other hand, estrogen may protect against heart disease. Clearly, women who are at high risk of developing breast cancer may want to avoid wine and drink red grape juice instead, while those women who are at risk of developing heart disease may want to add wine to their diet.

It is possible to have too much of a good thing. Although a glass or two of red wine daily may be beneficial, more than that can be harmful. In addition, some people should avoid wine altogether, notably those with liver problems or those taking prescription medications that should not be mixed with alcohol.

Sesame Oil and Seeds
Can prevent growth of tumors
Boost vitamin E

Sesame seed oil is often used in Asian cooking to add flavoring. Sesame seeds, either toasted or raw, add crunch and a subtle, nutty flavor to food.

Animal studies have shown that sesamin, an ingredient found in sesame oil, can inhibit the growth of cancerous tumors and can also lower cholesterol. Recently, sesamin has been shown to recycle vitamin E in the antioxidant network, making it an antioxidant booster. Sesamin also contains phytic acid, a potent antioxidant.

Sesame seeds and sesame oil are not only healthy but delicious. If you have not used these ingredients before, now is a great time to expand your culinary horizons. For a true phytochemical feast, sprinkle a few drops of sesame oil on lightly steamed vegetables, and top with sautéed sesame seeds.

Soy Foods
Protect against prostate and breast cancer
Lower cholesterol

Japan has the longest life span of any nation, as well as the lowest rate of heart disease in the world for women and the second-lowest rate for men. In addition, cancers that are common in the West, such as breast cancer and prostate cancer, are relatively rare in Japan. American women are four times more likely to die of breast cancer than Japanese women, and American men are five times more likely to die of prostate cancer than Japanese men.

To what can the Japanese attribute their good health? For one thing, the Japanese diet is much lower in fat and higher in fiber than the typical Western diet, but there is another striking difference: soybeans. Traditional Japanese cuisine is rich in a variety of foods derived from soy, including tofu or bean curd, tempeh (fermented soybean patty), miso (fermented bean paste), and edame (steamed, raw green soybeans). What is unique about soybeans is that they contain many disease-fighting phytochemicals that are not found in foods normally consumed in the West.

Soy is rich in isoflavones, a type of flavonoid that is special because it is converted in the body into phytoestrogens, very weak hormone-like compounds that may help to prevent hormone-dependent cancers such as breast and prostate cancer (these cancers are called hormone-dependent because hormones can stimulate their growth). Isoflavones bind to sites on cell membranes that are normally reserved for more harmful hormones that can stimulate the growth of tumors. Since these more potent hormones have no place to go, they are eliminated from the body before they can cause trouble.

Soy is the only food source of an isoflavone called *genistein,* which is being studied as a potential treatment for cancer. Genistein can inhibit the action of enzymes that promote cell growth and migration and can lead to the growth of tumors. Genistein blocks the growth of prostate cancer cells and breast cancer cells grown in tissue culture dishes.

Genistein's role as a cancer fighter has been widely studied. Interestingly, autopsies of Japanese men have shown that their rate of prostate cancer is as high as it is for American men, but the difference seems to be that the cancers grow much more slowly. In Japanese men, prostate tumors remain so small that the disease often does not progress to the point where the men develop any clinical symptoms of prostate cancer.

Recently, researchers compared the level of isoflavones in the blood plasma of American men with that of Japanese men, and what they found was astonishing. Japanese men had isoflavone levels that were 100 times higher than American men, and the primary isoflavone in their blood was genistein. Although more research needs to be done before we can conclusively say that soy foods protect against cancer, it seems likely that they do.

There is yet another reason to eat soy foods—they can lower high blood cholesterol levels. According to an analysis of thirty-eight studies undertaken by Dr. James Anderson of the University of Kentucky, eating a small amount of soy protein daily (the amount in 3 to 4 ounces of tofu) can dramatically lower elevated blood cholesterol and triglyceride levels. In addition, isoflavones, along with other antioxidants in soy, such as phytic acid, can also prevent the oxidation of LDL cholesterol, which can lead to clogged arteries.

Fortunately, as the good news about soy has become better known, there are many easy-to-use soy products on the market, such as soy burgers, soy shakes, and flavored soy milk. Soy sauce may be very tasty, but it does not contain isoflavones. Eat your soy!

Spinach
May prevent macular degeneration
Good source of folic acid

As some of you who watched cartoons as children may recall, whenever Popeye needed to pump up his muscles, he would down a can of spinach. Today we have scientific proof that spinach is indeed a power food—not for better muscles, but for better vision.

Raw spinach contains high amounts of lutein, a carotenoid that may have a strong protective effect against macular degeneration. A study conducted at five eye research centers in the United States showed that people who consumed the most lutein in their diet had a much lower incidence of macular degeneration than those who did not. Spinach was found to have a protective effect against this leading cause of blindness.

Spinach is one of the few food sources of lipoic acid, a network antioxidant. It is also an excellent source of the B vitamin folic acid, which is not an antioxidant, but which can nevertheless help prevent both heart disease and cancer. Folic acid is particularly important for women. Low levels of folic acid have been linked to an increased risk of both cervical cancer and birth defects.

Folic acid helps to maintain normal levels of homocysteine, an amino acid found in the body. In a study performed at Harvard Medical School, men with even slightly elevated levels of homocysteine were three times more likely to have heart attacks than those with normal levels. Elevated blood levels of homocysteine are now a recognized risk factor for cardiovascular disease.

Sweet Potatoes
Fight cancer
Protect your heart

One of the main points of *The Antioxidant Miracle* is just how easy it is to boost your intake of antioxidants simply by making the right food choices. Potatoes are a case in point. White potatoes are a terrific source of potassium and fiber but contain only a tiny amount of two antioxidants, lipoic acid and vitamin C. On the other hand, one medium-size baked sweet potato offers about 24,700 I.U. of retinol equivalents (from beta carotene or carotenoids), or five times the RDA for vitamin A, in addition to potassium and fiber. In fact, sweet potatoes are a better choice in terms of maintaining the antioxidant advantage than white potatoes. This doesn't mean that you shouldn't eat white potatoes, but it does mean that you should be eating sweet potatoes on many days other than Thanksgiving.

Tomatoes
Protect against prostate and stomach cancer

Have a slice or two of pizza. How about a heaping bowl of spaghetti marinara? Both are wonderful sources of lycopene, a carotenoid found in tomatoes that may protect against cancer and heart disease. In particular, lycopene appears to offer special protection against prostate cancer. Out of seven studies, five strongly associated a diet rich in lycopene with a significantly lower incidence of prostate cancer. In particular, lycopene protected against the most advanced and severe forms of prostate cancer.

Lycopene is not for men only. There is evidence that it can also benefit women. Even before the lycopene-prostate study, researchers examined the carotenoid intake of 102 women with precancerous conditions of the cervix and the same number of cancer-free women. They found that the women with the highest intake of lycopene had only one-fifth the risk of getting the precancerous condition as compared to those with the lowest intake. According to these researchers, the difference between low and high intake of lycopene was as little as eating one tomato a day.

Cooked tomatoes are a better source of lycopene than raw ones. My colleagues Helmut Sies and Willy Stahl have found that lycopene in tomato paste is better utilized by the body than that in whole tomatoes.

Since lycopene is fat-soluble, it is best absorbed by the body when eaten at mealtime with a bit of oil or cheese.

Lycopene is not the only cancer-fighting compound found in tomatoes. Tomatoes also contain *p*-coumaric acid and chlorogenic acid, which can block the formation of nitrosamines, cancer-causing compounds that are formed during normal digestion. (Vitamin C can also block nitrosamine formation.) Nitrosamines are dangerous because they can destroy DNA, which can lead to cancerous changes in cells. Nitrosamines occur when nitrites, a commonly used food preservative, or nitrates, a naturally occurring chemical in food, combine with amino acids. Nitrites are added to cured meats such as bacon, ham, pepperoni, or hot dogs as a coloring agent and to prevent botulism. If possible, try to avoid foods with added nitrites.

Watermelon and pink grapefruit are other sources of lycopene, although not as good as tomatoes.

Tea
Clears out clogged arteries
Reduces risk of many different types of cancer
Tea is not only the world's most popular beverage, it is also one of the world's healthiest. Don't confuse real tea with herbal teas made from a variety of different plants; real tea is made from the tea plant *(Camellia sinensis),* an evergreen that has been used for this purpose for about 6,000 years. Legend has it the first cup of tea was brewed by accident around 2735 B.C. when the leaves from a tea plant fell into boiling water at a reception held by the Chinese emperor Shen Nung. Tea became a favorite drink among the Chinese nobility, and the custom of tea drinking quickly spread throughout Asia.

There are three kinds of tea made from the tea plant: green tea, oolong, and black tea. When the tea leaves are processed or fermented, the leaves darken and develop a stronger flavor. Green tea, which is more lightly processed than the other varieties, is favored in Japan. The Chinese prefer oolong tea, which is partially fermented. In Europe and the West, black tea, which is fully fermented, is the most popular. All types of tea contain antioxidant flavonoids called polyphenols, which are also present in red wine. Although all forms of tea have proven health benefits, the polyphenols in green tea are believed to be more potent than those found in other teas.

Numerous studies report that tea drinkers of any variety have a lower risk of heart disease rate than those who don't drink tea. In all likelihood, the polyphenols in tea prevent the oxidation of LDL cholesterol, which can lead to artery-clogging plaque. They also enhance the antioxidant network by regenerating vitamin C. In a study conducted in the Netherlands, researchers examined the diets of 805 men aged sixty to eighty-four. The men who consumed the diet highest in flavonoids in general and tea in particular had a lower risk of having a fatal heart attack than those who drank tea infrequently or not at all. Follow-up studies have shown that men who drink the most tea also have the lowest risk of stroke.

Tea also appears to offer powerful protection against many different types of cancer, including colon, esophageal, pancreatic, lung, and skin. Both test tube and animal studies show that tea can inhibit the action of many carcinogens and slow down the growth of tumors. A recent Japanese study showed that women who drank the most green tea—as many as ten cups daily—had a significantly reduced risk of developing cancer compared to women who did not drink tea.

I'm not suggesting that you drink ten cups of tea daily, but even a cup or two may help to reduce your cancer risk when combined with an antioxidant-rich diet.

Tea contains only half the caffeine of a brewed cup of coffee. Nevertheless, if you're caffeine-sensitive, you may want to restrict your intake of caffeinated tea, especially at night. Although studies performed on decaffeinated tea showed that it offered health benefits, it had a weaker effect than caffeinated tea.

Turmeric
Protects against cancer

Turmeric is the spice that gives curry powder its golden yellow color. A member of the ginger family, the underground stem or root of the turmeric plant is dried and ground and used as both a flavoring and a preservative. Known as the "spice of life" since ancient times, turmeric has been used both in cooking and as a medicinal plant in India. In Ayurvedic, the Indian system of traditional medicine, turmeric has been used to promote good digestion, fight infection, treat liver problems, and relieve arthritis.

Long before the discovery of refrigeration, curry powder was used to preserve food that would get rancid if exposed to oxygen. Scientists have recently discovered that turmeric contains phenolic compounds that have antioxidant properties. They called these compounds *curcuminoids*. Several Indian studies show that curcuminoids can lower blood cholesterol levels and reduce inflammation. One double-blind study showed that curcuminoids worked as well in relieving pain and stiffness in arthritis patients as a prescription nonsteroidal anti-inflammatory medication. In addition, curcuminoids can inhibit the formation of many different types of cancers in animals exposed to known carcinogens. Similar to both ginkgo biloba and Pycnogenol, which also contain phenolic compounds, curcuminoids help to modulate the effects of nitric oxide that is produced by immune cells and can be harmful. Add a little turmeric—it tastes good, too.

Walnuts

Walnuts are an excellent source of cancer-fighting ellagic acid, but that's not all. These delicious nuts are high in heart-healthy monounsaturated fatty acids. Studies have shown that compared to low-fat diets or diets rich in corn oil, walnut oil can lower total cholesterol levels without raising blood triglyceride levels. Walnut oil can be used instead of olive oil to make a terrific salad dressing with raspberry vinegar. It can also be used in cooking.

Winter Squashes

Reduce risk of cataracts

Protect against heart disease

In the beginning of this chapter, I advised you to eat a variety of fruits and vegetables and, in particular, to look for those with the deepest, strongest colors. Here is a prime example. There are many different types of squash, but when it comes to antioxidant power, only the bright orange and yellow winter squash pack a punch.

Summer squash contains only trace amounts of carotenoids, but pumpkin contains a hefty amount of both alpha and beta carotene and a small quantity of lutein and zeaxanthin. Other varieties of winter squash contain high amounts of beta carotene as well as other beneficial minerals such as potassium and calcium.

The payoff for eating winter squash may be better vision. A twelve-year study of nurses conducted by researchers at Harvard University showed that those who ate the most fruits and vegetables rich in beta carotene had the lowest incidence of cataracts. Foods such as winter squash, spinach, and sweet potatoes offered the strongest protection.

An antioxidant-rich diet is an important first step in helping to maintain the antioxidant advantage, but it can't do the job alone. Daily supplementation with key antioxidants is another crucial step in fulfilling the Antioxidant Miracle. In the next chapter, you will learn which supplements you should be taking, how to take them, and how much to take.

14

The Packer Plan
Your Supplement Regimen

Our new understanding of the antioxidant network makes it easier than ever to enjoy the full benefits of the Antioxidant Miracle. By fortifying our antioxidant network with food and supplements, it is possible for us all to live longer, healthier lives free of many of the common diseases that have become associated with "normal" aging.

There is nothing normal about disease. Disease is most often the result of an abnormal environment inside and outside the body. Man-made hazards, such as pollution, cigarette smoke, alcohol abuse, and a nutrient-poor diet, have robbed us of the antioxidant advantage nature intended for us to have and are responsible for many common diseases, from heart disease to cancer to diabetes. Although these ailments strike later in life, their seeds are sown decades earlier.

In this chapter, I will show you how simple it is to regain your antioxidant advantage simply by taking the right combination of supplements. It is an easy and highly effective way to ensure that you are getting enough antioxidant protection.

First, I will recommend a basic antioxidant regimen that is designed to boost your network antioxidants to optimal levels. My program consists of several key network antioxidants and Antioxidant Boosters. My recommended doses are based on the latest scientific studies, which show how antioxidants work within the body. Some people may recommend higher doses of specific antioxidants; I, however, do not believe that more is necessarily better. Although I believe that the RDAs for antioxidants are ridiculously low, this does not mean that I endorse megadoses of supplements. There is no point in taking a supplement if it is not absorbed by the body. Therefore, my doses are carefully designed to naturally boost the level of network antioxidants in a safe, effective way.

Of course, not everybody is the same, and some people may require additional supplements. For that reason, I have also modified my basic program to accommodate people with special needs, such as diabetics, people at high risk of developing heart disease or stroke, smokers, people with a family history of cancer, athletes, postmenopausal women, and "picky eaters" who do not get enough antioxidants from food.

The basic network antioxidant cocktail

The basic network antioxidant cocktail described below uses standard products that you can find almost anywhere that supplements are sold. The dosages per capsule will vary from manufacturer to manufacturer, and you may need to adjust the capsule count accordingly, but the examples I have given below are fairly standard.

For your convenience, I recommend that you take your supplements in two doses: one in the morning and the other in the evening. (Some people find that if they take too many supplements at one time, they get an upset stomach.) Try to take your supplements with food for maximum absorption and to avoid any stomach problems. You can wash down your supplements with either water or juice.

If you find that it is easier for you to take more supplements in the morning than at night, that's fine. In most cases, it doesn't matter when you take your supplements, but there are two exceptions: vitamin C and lipoic acid. Both of these supplements are used by the body rapidly and need to be replenished within a few hours.

In addition to the antioxidant network and boosters, I have also added folic acid, a B vitamin, to the Packer Plan. As many of you may already know, folic acid has recently been discovered to protect against heart disease, cancer, and birth defects. Folic acid helps to maintain normal levels of homocysteine. The combination of folic acid and the network antioxidants should offer powerful protection against these and other common health problems.

Many of you may already be taking a multivitamin every day containing the RDA for a variety of vitamins and minerals. Since about 10 percent of the population is deficient in one micronutrient or another, a multivitamin is a good way to make sure that you are covering all of your nutritional bases. These multivitamins, however, typically do not contain a significant amount of antioxidants. Simply take the Packer Plan along with your multivitamin.

Some of you, however, may be taking high-potency multivitamins with high doses of antioxidants well beyond the RDA, and in many cases, higher than I recommend. In addition, the antioxidants in the multivitamins may not be in the optimal form. (For example, I recommend only natural vitamin E, and many multivitamins include synthetic vitamin E.) Therefore, if you go on the Packer Plan, discontinue taking a high-potency multivitamin. Instead, you can switch to a multivitamin that adheres to the RDAs.

Do not take a multivitamin that includes iron unless advised to do so by your physician. High levels of iron have been associated with an increased risk of heart disease.

The supplements listed on the following pages are available individually in the doses that I recommend from many manufacturers. The company that supplies formulations for our clinical trials will offer custom formulations of the Network Antioxidant Cocktail and Booster Packs through the web site at www.networkantioxidants.com. These products may be ordered directly from the toll-free number: 877-ANTIOXI or 877-268-4694. These custom formulations are not only more economical than purchasing each product separately, but they virtually halve the number of pills you need to take daily.

The basic antioxidant cocktail

Your A.M. Supplement Regimen

The Vitamin E Family
(1) 100 mg tocotrienols
(1) 200 mg mixed tocopherols

Co Q10
(1) 30 mg Co Q10

Lipoic Acid
(1) 50 mg lipoic acid

Vitamin C
(1) 250 mg ester vitamin C

Folic Acid
(1) 400 mcg folic acid

Biotin
(1) 300 mcg biotin

Vitamin B$_6$
(1) 2 mg vitamin B$_6$

Your P.M. Supplement Regimen

The Vitamin E Family
(1) 200 mg natural
alpha tocopherol

Lipoic Acid
(1) 50 mg lipoic acid

Vitamin C
(1) 250 mg ester C

Ginkgo Biloba
(1) 30 mg ginkgo
biloba

Selenium
(1) 200 mcg selenium

Special instructions

Select the Best Vitamin E

I recommend that you purchase three different types of vitamin E: natural alpha tocopherol, mixed tocopherols, and tocotrienols. As I discuss extensively in the chapter on vitamin E, each of these members of the vitamin E family is essential for health.

When you buy alpha tocopherol, be sure that the label specifies it is *natural* alpha tocopherol. You may have to read the fine print to know for sure what you are buying. Naturally derived vitamin E is always described as "*d*-alpha tocopherol." Synthetic vitamin E is properly labeled as "*dl*-alpha tocopherol." There is only a one-letter difference in labeling, but in my opinion, there is a big difference in terms of the quality of the product.

Natural vitamin E is a plant-derived form of the molecule as nature designed it and as is preferred by the human body. Synthetic vitamin E is a petroleum-based product that is not identical or functionally equivalent to natural vitamin E. Synthetic vitamin E is not harmful in normal dosages and, in fact, is also beneficial, but I do not believe it is as potent or effective as the natural variety.

Tocotrienols and mixed tocopherols are only sold in their natural form, so this is not an issue for these supplements.

What You Need to Know about Lipoic Acid

Lipoic acid is known by a variety of names, including thiotic acid, alpha lipoic acid, and 1,2 dithiolane-3-pentanoic acid. For purposes of simplicity, I have used the most commonly used name, lipoic acid—you may, however, see products sold in health food stores and pharmacies under other names, such as alpha lipotene or alphabetic.

Lipoic acid, which is part of the basic antioxidant cocktail, is a molecular cousin to the B vitamin biotin. They have a similar shape and are both known to improve insulin resistance in animals and humans. Unfortunately, these cousins don't get along. Lipoic acid can compete with biotin and, in the long run, interfere with biotin's activities in the body. To remedy this problem, I recommend taking biotin supplements when the daily intake of lipoic acid exceeds 100 milligrams as in my recommendations for smokers, diabetics, and people who may have a strong family history of cancer.

Select the Best Vitamin C

Vitamin C is sold in two forms—ascorbic acid and the mineral salt of ascorbic acid known as ester C. Although both forms of vitamin C are fine, ascorbic acid can increase the production of stomach acid, which can not only cause discomfort but can increase the absorption of iron from food. Since iron overload is a major risk factor for heart disease, it is advisable for most people to avoid excess iron.

Special boost for special needs

Cigarette Smokers and Secondhand Smokers

Cigarette smokers are a group with much to gain from antioxidant supplementation. Every time you inhale cigarette smoke, you are eroding your antioxidant defenses.

Cigarette smoke is a toxic soup that contains carbon monoxide, nitrogen dioxide, and carcinogenic tars. The tars overload the glutathione system. Smokers' systems need boosting with additional lipoic acid. Therefore, I recommend that smokers and people who are exposed to high levels of secondhand smoke add the following four additional supplements to the Packer Plan.

Smokers: In addition to the basic Packer Plan, add the following to either your A.M. or P.M. regimen.

(1) 100 mg lipoic acid
(1) 100 mg tocotrienols
(1) 50 mg Co Q10
(1) 20 mg Pycnogenol

Caution: Smokers should not take beta carotene or a carotenoid complex, since these compounds may interact negatively with cigarette smoke. They should eat a diet rich in fruits and vegetables.

Diabetics

About 20 percent of all Americans have some degree of insulin resistance, the first stage of adult-onset diabetes. Insulin resistance is often linked to impaired glucose tolerance. If you have been diagnosed with either insulin resistance or impaired glucose tolerance, I recommend that you add three additional supplements to your regimen: gamma linolenic acid (GLA, also known as evening primrose oil), chromium, and extra lipoic acid. You can add them to your morning or evening regimen.

GLA, an essential fatty acid that is usually manufactured in the body from an enzyme, helps to protect against heart disease. Diabetics lack this important enzyme and therefore need to take GLA supplements.

Chromium, a trace mineral, works with insulin to help the body utilize sugar and metabolize fat. Studies performed by the USDA show that chromium can help improve glucose tolerance, which is extremely beneficial for diabetics.

Diabetics: In addition to the basic Packer Plan, add the following to either your A.M. or P.M. regimen.

- (1) 100 mg lipoic acid
- (1) 1,000-mg GLA capsule
- (1) 200 mcg chromium

Athletes

As I have explained earlier, strenuous exercise puts your body under high levels of oxidative stress, which in the long run can damage muscle. The Packer Plan should provide enough antioxidants to protect and restore your antioxidant advantage. In addition, however, I recommend that you add an amino acid, L-carnitine, to your supplement regimen. L-carnitine is synthesized in the brain, heart, and skeletal muscles but may be needed in higher amounts in athletes. It transports fatty acids across the cell wall to the mitochondria, the powerhouse within the cell, providing the raw material needed to produce ATP, the body's fuel. Thus, it also functions as an antioxidant booster.

Athletes: In addition to the basic Packer Plan, add the following to either your A.M. or P.M. regimen.

- (1) 250 mg of L-carnitine

Menopausal Women

Postmenopausal women need additional calcium and should combine the basic cocktail with a calcium supplement. Test tube studies have shown that tocotrienols can offer protection against the kind of breast cancer that is most common after menopause. Therefore, I also recommend adding more tocotrienols to your antioxidant cocktail.

Postmenopausal women: In addition to the basic Packer Plan, add the following to either your A.M. or P.M. regimen.

- (1) 1,200 mg calcium
- (1) 100 mg tocotrienols

People at High Risk of Cancer

If you have a strong family history of cancer, that is, a primary relative (a parent, sibling, or grandparent) who died before the age of sixty of cancer, you may be at greater risk of developing it.

In most cases, you may not inherit a gene for a specific type of cancer, but rather a weakness in the genes that control the body's natural enzyme detoxification system. This means that over time, your body will lose its ability to fight carcinogens, leaving you vulnerable to many different types of cancer.

A family history of cancer is not a sentence of doom, but it does mean that you should limit your exposure to known carcinogens, particularly cigarette smoke. Get regular medical checkups: Early detection is important.

The basic Packer Plan will help maintain the body's antioxidant defenses, which work in tandem with the detoxification system to control the negative effects of carcinogens. In addition to the basic network antioxidant cocktail, I recommend that you take additional lipoic acid to further boost your levels of glutathione, the antioxidant that has an essential role in the detoxification process.

If you are at high risk of developing cancer: In addition to the basic Packer Plan, add the following to either your A.M. or P.M. regimen.

  (1) 100 mg lipoic acid
  (1) 100 mg tocotrienols
  (1) 50 mg Co Q10
  (1) 20 mg Pycnogenol

People at High Risk of Cardiovascular Disease

A family history of cardiovascular disease—if your mother died before age fifty or your father died before age sixty of heart disease—you are considered to be at high risk of having a heart attack or stroke. There is very strong evidence that antioxidants in general, and vitamin E and Co Q10 in particular, can greatly reduce your risk. This book is replete with studies confirming the link between a high intake of vitamin E and a reduced risk of heart disease. Similarly, the effects of Co Q10 in preventing heart failure are well documented.

I am particularly proud of the Packer Lab's contribution in showing how network antioxidants can minimize the damage of reperfusion injury after a heart attack or stroke.

There are many people who may be at risk of stroke and not even know it. People with untreated high blood pressure are particularly vulnerable to stroke, as are those who have been diagnosed with carotid stenosis, the blockage of the arteries in the neck that deliver blood to the brain. These problems typically do not produce any symptoms; the only way you would know that you have them is if they were detected during a physical exam. Be vigilant about seeing your doctor at least once a year for a thorough checkup. If your doctor has prescribed warfarin or other blood-thinning medications, be sure to tell him or her that you are taking antioxidants. Network antioxidants are natural anticoagulants; therefore, your doctor may wish to revise your prescription.

If you are at high risk of developing heart disease or have a family history of stroke or a medical condition that can lead to stroke, particularly high blood pressure, add the following to either your A.M. or P.M. regimen in addition to the basic Packer Plan.

(1) 50 mg Co Q10 (A.M. or P.M.)
(1) 100 mg tocotrienols (P.M.)
(1) 100 mg lipoic acid
(1) 20 mg Pycnogenol

Picky Eaters

You know who you are! If just the thought of eating broccoli makes you weak in the knees, and if drinking a glass of orange juice daily is a challenge, you need to enhance your antioxidant intake by taking your fruits and vegetables in a pill. I believe that there is no substitute for a good diet, but there are new supplements on the market that come close to duplicating some of Mother Nature's best creations (such as products offered by Golden Neolife Diamite International).

Flavonoid complex contains a mixture of important components from green tea; cranberry; kale; beet; mixed berry; red and black grapes; orange, lemon, and grapefruit extracts.

Cruciferous-plus contains a mixture of important compounds extracted from broccoli, radish, black mustard, watercress, licorice root, kale, and other important members of this illustrious cancer-fighting family.

Carotenoid complex contains a mixture of important compounds extracted from fruits and vegetables such as tomato, carrot, spinach, red bell pepper, strawberry, apricot, and peach.

Picky eaters: Add these supplements to your regimen daily, either morning or evening.

(1) Flavonoid complex
(1) Cruciferous-plus
(1) Mixed carotenoid complex

Caution for smokers: Smokers often neglect to eat enough fruits and vegetables, but even so, they should avoid taking supplementary carotenoids. Flavonoid complex and cruciferous-plus are fine for smokers.

Questions and answers about the Packer Plan

Now that I have given specific information on which supplements you should be taking, I will answer some questions I am often asked about antioxidant supplements.

WHERE SHOULD I BUY MY SUPPLEMENTS?   Gone are the days when supplements were only sold in a handful of health food stores. Today, high-quality supplements can be found in pharmacies, discount stores, catalogs, on the Internet, and of course, in the literally thousands of health food stores and natural food supermarkets across the nation. My advice is to buy your supplements wherever it is most economical and convenient. Prices vary widely on supplements, so watch for sales. Frequently, some of the larger health food stores and pharmacies have two-for-one sales, which can provide substantial savings.

WHICH BRANDS ARE THE BEST?   Generally, the same rules apply to buying supplements that apply to buying any over-the-counter medication: Select products offered by reputable manufacturers that take special steps to ensure safety and effectiveness. Be sure to buy products that come in tamper-proof packages, preferably with an inside and outside safety seal. It is also advisable to purchase products that are marked with an expiration date.

To maintain the quality of the products you buy, store them in a cool, dry area out of direct sunlight.

WHAT FORMS OF SUPPLEMENTS ARE THE MOST EFFECTIVE?   Supplements come in many different forms, from pills to tablets to capsules to creams that are absorbed through the skin. There are even powders that can be mixed in juice or water for people who are unable to swallow pills. Unless I specify otherwise, choose the form that is easiest for you to use.

CAN I COMBINE SUPPLEMENTS WITH PRESCRIPTION MEDICATION?
Usually, it is safe to take most supplements with prescription medication, but there are exceptions. For example, vitamin E and ginkgo biloba are natural blood thinners and, therefore, should not be taken along with a prescription blood thinner such as Coumadin.

Diabetics take note: If you are taking medication for diabetes, be sure to tell your doctor that you are also taking antioxidants. Although antioxidants will be of great benefit to diabetics, vitamin C can skew the results of blood sugar tests. Accordingly, patients should inquire whether their doctor would prefer that they abstain from taking their antioxidants for twenty-four hours before being tested.

The rule of thumb is, if you are using prescription medication, check with your doctor to make sure that it is not interfering with your medicine.

WHAT DO THE DOSAGE NUMBERS MEAN? Antioxidants are micronutrients, which means that you only need to ingest a comparatively small amount to get maximum benefit. There are two kinds of antioxidants: water-soluble and fat-soluble. Water-soluble antioxidants are not stored in the body and are excreted in urine. Fat-soluble antioxidants are stored in fatty tissue.

Water-soluble antioxidants are usually measured in either milligrams (mg), which are equal to $\frac{1}{1000}$ of a gram, or micrograms (mcg), which are equal to $\frac{1}{1,000,000}$ of a gram.

Fat-soluble antioxidants may be measured in either mg or mcg or in I.U. (international units). Basically, 1 I.U. is equal to 1 mg.

IF MAINTAINING AN OPTIMAL LEVEL OF NETWORK ANTIOXIDANTS IS KEY TO ACHIEVING GOOD HEALTH, CAN MY DOCTOR CHECK MY ANTIOXIDANT LEVEL TO TRACK MY PROGRESS? Yes, there is a simple blood test called the *Pantox Profile*, which can measure antioxidant levels in your body, as well as levels of other key indicators of health. A blood sample taken at your doctor's office is sent to Pantox Laboratories in San Diego where it is analyzed. A comprehensive report is later sent to your doctor.

Designed by a group of research scientists (myself included), this test not only measures the levels of the network antioxidants but also provides detailed information on twenty different substances found in serum, including cholesterol, iron, glucose, and homocysteine levels. (Homocysteine is the amino acid that in high amounts has been associated with an increased risk of heart disease and cancer.) The Pantox Profile will determine whether your levels of antioxidants fall within the optimal, average, or poor range.

In most cases, if you are following the Packer Plan, you will have an excellent Pantox Profile. In rare cases, however, because of biochemical variations, some people may not be able to absorb supplements as well as others. Therefore, these people may require higher than normal doses of particular antioxidants and may have to make dietary adjustments.

The Pantox Profile costs around $300 and may be covered by some insurance policies. Although testing for antioxidant levels is not widely practiced today, I believe that in the near future, having your levels of antioxidants checked will be as routine a part of your annual physical as having your cholesterol levels measured.

If you want to see what a Pantox Profile looks like, turn to Appendix A, page 208.

15

The Packer Plan
Antioxidants for Healthy, Beautiful Skin

The Antioxidant Miracle not only works on the inside of your body, it can have an even more dramatic effect on the outside. Maintaining the antioxidant advantage will not just keep you in good health but will keep you looking good.

Every cell of your body needs antioxidants, and the cells in your skin are no exception. The skin is the one of the hardest-working organ systems in the body, a fact that may come as a surprise to those of you who think of the skin merely as a protective covering.

In reality, your skin plays a far more important role in the body than merely a cosmetic one. It is vital to your health. The skin is your first line of defense against viruses, bacteria, fungi, and foreign invaders. It enables the body to retain fluids, which are essential for life and for the maintenance of body temperature. Skin is also instrumental for the production and storage of vitamin D, which is necessary for the absorption of calcium.

Your skin is also the organ system that is most vulnerable to free radical attack, for obvious reasons. It is constantly exposed to sunlight and pollutants such as ozone, which promote the formation of free

197

radicals. Cigarette smoke, which is teeming with free radicals, is a major culprit of skin aging. Smokers often have wrinkles equivalent to people ten years their senior, not to mention sallow, gray skin.

In fact, because we often don't protect ourselves adequately against these environmental assaults, we are not only aging our skin more rapidly than need be, but we are making ourselves more prone to skin cancer. As you will see, the most effective way to prevent both skin aging and skin cancer is to maintain the antioxidant advantage, not only on the inside of your body, but on the outside as well.

Regardless of external environmental stressors, there are particular changes that occur to our skin as part of the natural aging process. Skin consists of various layers. The epidermal surface is the outer layer that is visible to the eye; the dermis is the underlying layer we cannot see. The epidermis consists of cells that are mature and ready to be replaced. Young skin typically has a fresh, dewy glow because the outer epidermal cells are replaced rapidly. As we age, however, skin begins to look worn and dull, which is a reflection of the slowdown in the production of new cells.

Older skin not only looks more drab than younger skin, but it also begins to wrinkle and sag. This is caused by changes in the underlying dermis. The dermis is made primarily of collagen, a protein that provides the scaffolding that supports the outer epidermis. There is an age-related decline in collagen production, which creates gaps in the scaffolding that leads to wrinkles and fine lines.

At the same time, there is a gradual breakdown in the microcirculation: the tiny vessels delivering blood and nutrients to the skin cells do not work as efficiently. Therefore, the skin cells are not receiving adequate nourishment. To compound the problem, skin loses the cells that help it to maintain moisture, which dries out the skin.

These normal age-related changes alone, however, are subtle and occur over time. The most dramatic changes to skin—the kind that make us look years older than we need to—are caused by photoaging, or exposure to ultraviolet (UV) rays produced by the sun.

Compare the skin on your face to the skin on another part of your body that is rarely exposed to the sun, and you will see a dramatic difference. If you're like most people, the skin on your face will undoubtedly look older, have a rougher texture, and perhaps have wrinkles and age spots. But the skin on an area that is protected from the sun will be smooth, supple, and wrinkle-free. The difference is especially apparent among people who have spent a great deal of time working outdoors, but it is also true for those who sunbathe, relaxing at the beach or poolside.

Why does sunlight exact such a steep toll on our skin? There are two kinds of UV rays emitted from the sun: UVA and UVB. Known as the burning rays, the effects of UVB exposure are felt almost immediately. These rays penetrate the dermis and cause sunburn. Even if you tan, these rays are harmful. Although UVA rays do not readily cause sunburn, the rays penetrate deep into the dermal layer and even to the fat underneath. The fundamental problem is that both types of UV radiation trigger the formation of free radicals that can damage proteins, fats, and DNA. Damage from UV light is cumulative: it can take years before the damaging effects become apparent. Generally, by the time we reach our mid-thirties, the long-term effects of UV exposure start to become visible in the form of fine lines, wrinkles, and telltale changes in skin tone and color. In sum, both UVA and UVB can wreak havoc on skin.

It is no coincidence that the rate of skin cancer has been steadily rising in proportion to exposure to UV light, and our changing attitudes toward getting a suntan. At the turn of the century, when skin cancer was relatively rare, a suntan was considered the mark of someone who was forced to toil outdoors, and it was avoided by those who were in what were then considered more prestigious professions. By the 1950s, the growing popularity of airplane travel created a new generation of people who could afford to hop a plane in the dead of winter for a weekend in the sun and wanted everyone else to know. The telltale suntan became a status symbol. Numerous suntan lotion products were promoted as allowing you to get a "healthy tan" while protecting against the so-called bad burning rays. As we were to later discover, there is no such thing as a healthy suntan. Any discoloration of skin from the sun is a sign of injury. At the same time, pollutants in the environment were causing a wearing down of the ozone layer, which helped to filter out UV rays before they reached the Earth's surface. Not only were we basking in the sun for hours at a time, but we were exposing ourselves to even stronger sunlight.

Today, attitudes toward suntans have shifted yet again. We no longer use suntan lotion to promote tanning; rather, we try to protect our skin by using sunscreens and sunblocks to filter out UV rays. Sunscreens and sunblocks may help to prevent some signs of skin aging, such as wrinkles, and even some of the less serious forms of skin cancer, but they apparently have not been particularly effective against the most potentially dangerous form of skin cancer—melanoma.

Close to 1 million new cases of skin cancer were diagnosed this year, and it is the leading cancer among men. Although many cases of skin cancer can be successfully treated, melanoma can be deadly. The best way to avoid skin cancer is to limit exposure to the sun as much as possible.

Like other organ systems within the body, the skin is also protected against free radical attack by the antioxidant network. In the Packer Lab, we have performed several experiments that demonstrate the effect of UV radiation on the skin. After even a brief exposure to UV radiation, there is a rapid and dramatic depletion of key antioxidants such as vitamin E, Coenzyme Q10, vitamin C, glutathione, and the supporting antioxidant enzymes.

Most important, we have learned that the antioxidant defense network works the same outside the body as it does inside. The antioxidants in the skin can recycle each other the same way that they do within the body. We have also shown that the external application of antioxidants is a very effective way to support the entire antioxidant network. Although taking oral supplements will help to boost the amount of antioxidants in your skin, the direct application of antioxidants to the skin is a much faster way to increase the level of antioxidants. Since the face and neck are particularly vulnerable to skin aging, I recommend that you use a combination of antioxidant creams on these areas.

Bolstering the antioxidant network both on the inside and the outside of your body is the key to having healthy, youthful, and resilient skin. Although there is no way to completely prevent skin aging, it is well within our power to slow it down considerably. It is also possible to reverse some of the damage that has already been done.

LIMIT YOUR EXPOSURE TO THE SUN   Simply staying out of the sun during peak burning hours (late morning to midafternoon) is a good way to reduce your exposure to free radicals. As I noted earlier, wearing a sunblock or sunscreen does not offer blanket protection against cancer, but it will reduce the signs of skin aging. Once you reduce the amount of environmental stress on your skin, your skin will be able to expend more energy on healing and repairing itself. Keep in mind, however, that many sunscreens do not protect against UVA rays. Be sure whatever product you use offers full spectrum protection.

BOOST YOUR SKIN'S NATURAL ANTIOXIDANT DEFENSES   Replenishing antioxidants directly on your skin is a wonderful way to keep your skin healthy and youthful. There are three key antioxidants that are part of the Packer Plan's skin-care regimen: vitamin C, vitamin E, and Pycnogenol. These antioxidants work together to boost the entire antioxidant network within the skin, providing wonderful protection against free radicals. Optimal skin care requires that these three antioxidants be both taken orally and applied directly on the skin.

Fortunately, there are now numerous antioxidant skin-care products that are sold at pharmacies, department stores, and even health food stores. Unfortunately, many of the products that claim to have antioxidants don't have enough of the antioxidants to be beneficial. As a rule of thumb, look for a product in which the antioxidant is one of the first ingredients listed on the label. In some cases, the label will list the particular potency of the product.

Before using any skin product, test it on a small piece of skin to make sure that you are not allergic or sensitive to it. Place a small amount of cream on your upper arm and cover it with a Band-Aid. Wait twenty-four hours. If you do not develop an irritation, you can try it on your face.

Below I outline the Packer Plan's state-of-the-art skin-care regimen to help harness the power of antioxidants to revitalize your skin.

An antioxidant feast for your face

Topical Vitamin C and Your Skin

Vitamin C's primary job within the antioxidant network is to recycle vitamin E, which is important on the outside of the body as well as on the inside. But that's not the only reason why I recommend using vitamin C cream or serum on your face. Recent studies suggest that vitamin C applied externally to the skin may do what was once considered impossible: stimulate the growth of new collagen.

Vitamin C is essential for the production of new collagen, but as we age, there is a decline in the amount of available vitamin C in the skin. As noted earlier, when taken orally, most of the antioxidant supplements are used within the cells of the body, and do not get delivered to skin cells. Several studies show that high-potency vitamin C creams (with over 10 percent concentration of vitamin C) can increase the level of this important vitamin in the skin. According to animal studies conducted at Duke University Medical Center, skin cells treated with vitamin C actually become thicker, which is a sign of collagen regeneration.

Applying vitamin C directly to the skin will help to restore skin tone, plump up wrinkles, and fill in small lines, giving skin a more youthful look. Topically applied vitamin C improves blood supply to the skin, giving the skin a more youthful glow. In addition, vitamin C creams and serums can minimize fine lines, reduce light wrinkles, and improve skin color and tone.

Vitamin C may also be able to protect skin from damage inflicted by UV light and to reduce some of the inflammation caused by UV exposure. Studies have shown that topically applied vitamin C can prevent one of the most dangerous effects of UV exposure: the suppression of the immune system. This means that vitamin C not only has a cosmetic effect but offers serious protection against further damage to the skin.

Vitamin C should only be used in specially formulated products designed specifically for external use. Look for products that contain a 10 percent concentration of vitamin C in a low pH, the form in which vitamin C is best absorbed by the skin. Vitamin C is available as a liquid serum or cream. Weaker versions of the serum and cream are designed to be used around the delicate eye area.

The serums are stronger than the creams and therefore are more effective. However, people with very sensitive skin may find them to be too irritating and may prefer to use a cream.

In the morning, after you wash your face, apply vitamin C cream or serum directly on the clean surface. Do not apply any moisturizers underneath; they will interfere with the absorption of the vitamin C.

Vitamin E and Your Skin

Vitamin E is one of the most important antioxidants in your skin; therefore, it is necessary to replenish it daily, inside and outside. The more you go outdoors, the more you need vitamin E. We have found that at a dose of UV light equal to about ten minutes of exposure to natural sunlight, there is a 50 percent reduction in the concentration of vitamin E in the skin. In animal studies, we have seen a surge in lipid hydro-peroxides (a sign of oxidative damage) in the skin immediately following exposure to UV light. We conducted two studies that clearly show the power of vitamin E to protect against damage to skin caused by UV exposure. In one study, we fed animals a diet supplemented with vitamin E. It took four weeks for the concentration of E in the skin to increase eightfold. When these mice were exposed to UV radiation, they experienced only one-third the rate of increase in lipid hydroperoxides that we saw in the unsupplemented mice. Vitamin E supplements reduced the damage by two-thirds.

But the even better news is that when we applied vitamin E cream directly to the skin of mice, the concentration of vitamin E soared ten- to twelvefold within a mere twenty-four hours. Not only that, when we exposed these mice to UV radiation similar to sunlight, there was a dramatic decrease in the telltale signs of oxidative damage.

A handful of studies suggest that vitamin E may also help reduce the signs of skin aging. In a study of twenty women between the ages of forty-two and sixty-four, over half showed a remarkable decrease in wrinkle amplitude and roughness on the eyelid treated with vitamin E cream daily for four weeks as opposed to the eyelid treated with a placebo cream. The researchers observed that the topical use of vitamin E cream helped smooth fine lines and wrinkles in sensitive areas of the face.

I recommend that you use a vitamin E–based cream at least once daily, preferably in the morning before you go outdoors and are exposed to the sun. I don't advise using the oil from a vitamin E capsule directly on your skin; it can cause irritation in some people. It is advisable to use a formulation of vitamin E cream specially designed for external application.

For best results, look for a cream or gel that contains vitamin E in the form of d-alpha-tocopherol rather than tocopheryl acetate or succinate, as these forms of vitamin E may not be directly available to skin cells.

For an added antioxidant boost

Remember: the best protecton is a combination of creams and serums applied externally and/or tablets taken orally. A complete program of network antioxidants has been formulated specifically to protect against skin aging. (See Appendix A, The Packer Plan.)

If your skin is showing obvious signs of aging, or you have a history of long-term exposure to the sun, I recommend that you take an extra 200 milligrams of tocotrienols daily in addition to the basic Packer Plan supplement regimen.

Pycnogenol Cream and Gel

In the antioxidant network, Pycnogenol enhances the action of vitamin C, another essential vitamin for youthful, glowing skin. It can be taken orally, or used externally on the skin. Rich in proanthocyanids and flavonoids, Pycnogenol contains more than forty antioxidants. There are several brands of skin creams and gels that include Pycnogenol, usually in combination with other antioxidants such as vitamin E (such as derma E). Pycnogenol helps maintain healthy, beautiful skin in several important ways. The flavonoids in Pycnogenol help to strengthen capillaries, the tiny blood vessels that deliver blood and nutrients to tissues and cells in your body, including those in the skin. As we age, these tiny capillaries begin to break down, resulting in diminished blood flow. Fortifying these tiny blood vessels will improve circulation throughout the body, including the skin.

As I mentioned earlier, older skin begins to sag and wrinkle because of the loss of collagen fibers. Studies have shown that Pycnogenol can help protect collagen against free radical attack, and even stimulate collagen repair. In one study, collagen fibers were soaked in water for twenty-four hours with a weight attached to them so that they would become weakened and stretched out. It's like adding decades of wear and tear to your skin overnight. However, when Pycnogenol was added to the water, the fibers actually shortened and became stronger, which in a sense was like rejuvenating skin.

Owing to its high antioxidant content, Pycnogenol also provides added protection against damaging UV rays. In one study performed in Finland, human skin cells were exposed to UV radiation. Without any protection and after prolonged exposure, about 50 percent of the skin cells died. However, when Pycnogenol was added to the cells, 85 percent of them survived the UV radiation. In particular, Pycnogenol can protect against dangerous UVB rays that are responsible for sunburns and damage to the outer layer of skin, the epidermis.

Pycnogenol is also a natural anti-inflammatory. I have heard numerous anecdotal reports that Pycnogenol gel is excellent on sensitive skin.

Apply Pycnogenol cream or gel over the vitamin E cream. After you have applied your antioxidants, you can use a moisturizer and apply your sunscreen or sunblock. If you wear makeup, apply it over your sun protection. Men can apply their antioxidant skin products at bedtime or after shaving.

The Packer Plan antioxidant skin-care regimen should not take more than five minutes each day, yet the benefits will be felt for decades to come. Our new knowledge of the causes of skin aging, combined with our understanding of how antioxidants work, now makes it possible to harness the power of antioxidants to maintain a lifetime of healthy, youthful skin.

Afterword: Toward a New Understanding of Health

When we look back on the spectacular accomplishments of the twentieth century, I have no doubt that the incredible advances we have made in medicine will be perceived as one of our crowning achievements, right along with landing a man on the moon and the invention of the computer chip.

Through better sanitation, antibiotics, vaccinations, and improved nutrition, we have added three decades to people's average life expectancy. The fastest-growing segment of the U.S. population is men and women aged seventy-five and older.

Yet it can be argued that we have learned as much from our mistakes as we have from our accomplishments. One of the primary lessons we have learned is that it can be pointless—and even cruel—to add years to life if there is no quality of life to those years. For many older people, life can become more of a burden than a joy.

Although we have paid lip service to preventive medicine, we have only just begun to take it seriously. Until recently, the underlying assumption was that a society that could conquer space and invent penicillin could handily defeat cancer, heart disease, and other common killers. Diet and lifestyle played second fiddle to dazzling, high-tech drugs that could be created in the laboratory. As many of us turned over our health care to the "experts," we were relegated to the role of bystanders.

Although we have an enormous arsenal of wonderful drugs and therapies that do indeed save lives, our entire approach to health care has been reactive as opposed to proactive. The system is designed to spring into action once a disease has taken hold, not before. Very often, by that time it is too late.

Unfortunately, many people are not spending their final decades enjoying life, but rather life is punctuated by visits to hospitals or doctors. The diseases of aging—diabetes, heart disease, arthritis, Alzheimer's disease, and cancer, among others—have exacted a steep toll on our quality of life.

Conventional, drug-oriented medicine may help us live longer, but it may not help us live better. My goal is not only to extend life, but to make later decades as vibrant and fulfilling as earlier decades.

Our growing knowledge of the antioxidant network now enables us, for the first time, to practice real preventive medicine. We now understand the role that free radicals play in the onset and progression of nearly every known disease, and more important, how they can be controlled by antioxidants. Simply by fortifying the body's antioxidant network, it is now possible to give the body the tools it needs to wage an effective fight against disease. Following the Packer Plan—eating an antioxidant-rich diet and taking the right supplements—can make a huge difference in whether we spend our last years playing tennis, sailing, or pursuing other meaningful activities, or being preoccupied with sickness and limited by physical infirmity.

The antioxidant network and its boosters offer new hope for preventing the epidemic of cancer and heart disease that devastates the lives of millions of Americans each year. Just as the discovery of penicillin changed the practice of medicine earlier in this century, the antioxidant network has the potential to create a new paradigm for health.

The power of the antioxidant network will be harnessed to treat many common diseases, often in combination with established medical therapies. The Packer Lab's recent discovery that antioxidants can regulate genes creates a world of possibilities: new drugs that work by bolstering the body's ability to fight against disease on its own, without the need for harsh, potentially dangerous drugs that often have unwanted side effects. In particular, I see antioxidants being used along with chemotherapy drugs in the treatment of cancer. I also predict that our knowledge of the relationship between antioxidants and genes will result in new drugs specifically tailored to quash bad genes before they can wreak havoc on the body. I have no doubt that there will come a day when breast cancer, prostate cancer, heart disease, and other common killers are controlled through our genes, and antioxidants will be very much involved in the process.

The Antioxidant Miracle gives us an opportunity to reclaim our health and, in a very real sense, our destinies. It enables us to take control over how well we age and makes the promise of a longer, healthier life.

Appendix A
Resources

The Packer Plan

For further information on the Packer Plan, or to order network antioxidant formulations, visit the web site at: networkantioxidants.com or phone toll-free 877-ANTIOXI (877-268-4694).

VERIS

The VERIS Research Information Service is a not-for-profit corporation that strives to provide a responsible source of information on the role of nutrition in health, with emphasis on the antioxidants, to health professionals, researchers, and health and nutrition educators/communicators worldwide. Additional information can be obtained on the worldwide web at: http://www.veris-online.org.

Saas Fee Declaration

In June 1992, I helped organize a meeting of seventeen of the world's leading scientists at the village of Saas Fee, Switzerland, where the air is crystal clear and the skiing is magnificent, even in June. In that idyllic environment, this group of researchers, who have dedicated their professional lives to studying antioxidant and free radical biology, examined and celebrated some startling new discoveries about the role of antioxidants and free radicals in the prevention and treatment of many chronic and degenerative diseases.

At the Saas Fee meeting, we studied the overwhelming body of evidence that shows that if used strategically, antioxidants can help maintain our health and vigor well into our seventh, eighth, and ninth decades, and perhaps even longer. With great excitement, we listened as our colleagues reported on groundbreaking research that will profoundly affect the way medicine will be practiced in the twenty-first century, which is right around the corner. Eager to generate greater scientific and public interest in the field of antioxidants, eight of the conference participants (including me) composed and affixed our signatures to a document we called "The Saas Fee Declaration." The essence of the declaration is that the scientific evidence that antioxidants play a pivotal role in maintaining health and preventing disease is now overwhelming and incontrovertible, and that scientists, health-care professionals, and the government have a duty to inform the public about this.

After the meeting, we circulated "The Saas Fee Declaration" among our colleagues around the world, and it has since been signed by hundreds of others. In fact, the response of the international scientific community has been so overwhelming that we've run out of room for signatures! I would like to share the "The Saas Fee Declaration" with you here so that you can begin to understand what the excitement is all about.

Saas Fee Declaration

ON THE SIGNIFICANCE OF ANTIOXIDANT NUTRIENTS IN PREVENTIVE MEDICINE

1. The intensive research on free radicals of the past fifteen years by scientists worldwide has led to the statement in 1992 that antioxidant nutrients may have major significance in the prevention of a number of diseases. These include cardiovascular and cerebrovascular disease, some forms of cancer, and several other disorders, many of which may be age-related.

2. There is now general agreement that there is a need for further work at the fundamental scientific level, as well as in large-scale randomized trials and in clinical medicine, which can be expected to lead to more precise information being made available.

3. The major objective of this work is the prevention of disease. This may be achieved by the use of antioxidants, which are natural physiological substances. The strategy should be to achieve optimal intakes of these antioxidant nutrients as part of preventive medicine.

4. It is quite clear that many environmental sources of free radicals exist, such as ozone, sunlight, and other forms of radiation, smog, dust, and other atmospheric pollutants. The optimal intake of antioxidants provides a preventive measure against these hazards.

5. There is a great need for improvement in public awareness of the potential preventive benefits of antioxidant nutrient intake. There is overwhelming evidence that the antioxidant nutrients such as vitamin E, vitamin C, carotenoids, alpha-lipoic acid, and others are safe even at very high levels of intake.

6. Moreover, there is now substantial agreement that governmental agencies, health professionals, and the media should promote information transfer to the general public, particularly when evidence exists that benefits for human health and public expenditure are overwhelming.

Igor Afanas`ev, Moscow
Julie E. Buring, Harvard
Anthony T. Diplock, London
Charles H. Hennekens, Harvard
Bodo Kuklinski, Rostock
Mathilde Maiorino, Padua
Lester Packer, Berkeley
Mulchand S. Patel, Cleveland
Karlheinz Schmidt, Tübingen

Appendix C

Sample Profiles

Explanation of a Poor Plasma Antioxidant Profile

Enclosed are the Pantox Profiles for your patient. Below are suggestions to you about his specific test results; they are not to be considered prescriptions for the patient or recommendations for the general population.

Following this, the test results are presented in a bar graph that compares each measured (or calculated) value with others in our database from individuals of the same sex and age. The very large Pantox database makes this possible.

THE LIPID-SOLUBLE ANTIOXIDANT PROFILE HAS FIVE COMPONENTS THAT NEED ATTENTION

* The Co Q10 value is low, falling in percentile 11. For adults, supplementation may be appropriate with an additional 25 milligrams, twice per day, because Q10 (and/or vitamin C) is necessary for vitamin E to exert its protective action.

* The vitamin E level is unusually low, falling in percentile 0. The consumption of an additional 4 to 8 I.U. per pound of body weight daily will generally increase the vitamin E level into the higher percentiles. The level of vitamin E is below the minimum shown by the studies of K. F. Gey and colleagues to be associated with higher risk.

* The gamma tocopherol level is moderate, falling in percentile 61. At present there are no supplements for this more active form of vitamin E, but it can be acquired by eating wheat germ, whole grains, and nuts.

Example of a Poor Plasma Antioxidant Profile

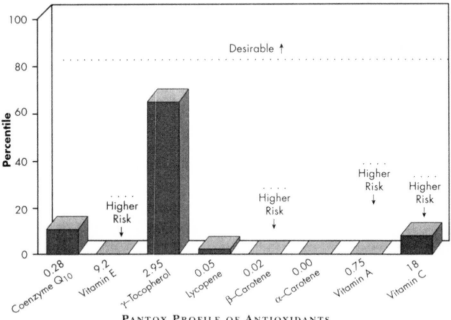

PANTOX PROFILE OF ANTIOXIDANTS

* The lycopene level is unusually low, falling in percentile 0. The consumption of tomatoes and tomato paste will generally increase these levels into the higher percentiles. Recent evidence suggests that this is a good idea.

* The beta carotene level is unusually low, falling in percentile 0. The consumption of fruits and colored vegetables will often increase these levels into the higher percentiles. There is overwhelming evidence that the consumption of fruits and vegetables promotes health and postpones diseases of many kinds. Specific supplementation with 25 mg/day of beta carotene would also be a suggested addition. The level of beta carotene is below the minimum shown by the studies of K. F. Gey and colleagues to be associated with higher risk.

* The alpha carotene level is unusually low, falling in percentile 0. A diet of fruits and colored vegetables is the only known source of this minor carotenoid. The low level could indicate a diet that is deficient in fruits and veggies.

* The vitamin A level is unusually low, falling in percentile 0. Vitamin A is essential for the immune response and is also involved in other defenses against infectious agents. Most people can increase their level of vitamin A by the consumption of 5,000 I.U./day of retinyl palmitate. Beta carotene can be converted to vitamin A, but in many individuals this conversion is slow and ineffectual. It is a good idea to have good levels of *both*.

* The lipid protection ratio (not shown) is unusually low, falling in percentile 0. This results mainly from a vitamin E value falling in percentile 0 and a cholesterol level falling in percentile 5. The easiest way to increase this ratio is to improve one's vitamin E level as described above. Lowering cholesterol is much harder to do. The lipid protection ratio is below the minimum shown by the studies of K. F. Gey and colleagues to be associated with higher risk.

To have your own Pantox Profile done, call them at 1-888-PANTOX8 (726-8698) or go to http://www.pantox.com.

Explanation of a Good Plasma Antioxidant Profile

THE LIPID-SOLUBLE ANTIOXIDANT PROFILE COULD BE IMPROVED

* The Co Q10 is an ideal range falling in percentile 74. No action is needed.

* The vitamin E level is excellent, falling in percentile 93. Further supplementation with vitamin E is not needed.

* The gamma tocopherol level is low, falling in percentile 10. At present there are no supplements for this more active form of vitamin E, but it can be acquired by eating wheat germ, whole grains, and nuts.

* The lycopene level is low, falling in percentile 28. The consumption of tomatoes and tomato paste will generally increase these levels into the higher percentiles. Recent evidence suggests that this is a good idea.

* The beta carotene level is excellent, falling in percentile 90. Further efforts to increase this level are not indicated.

Example of a Good Plasma Antioxidant Profile

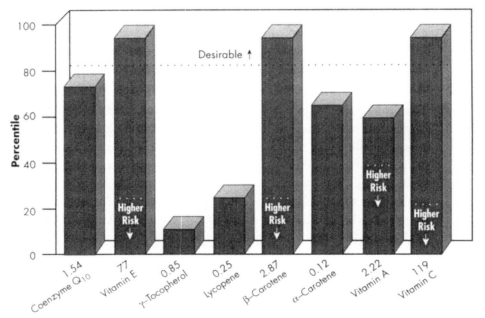

Pantox Profile of Antioxidants

* The alpha carotene level is moderate, falling in percentile 63. A diet of fruits and colored vegetables is the only known source of this minor carotenoid. This moderate level is an indication of a diet that includes some fruits and vegetables.

* The vitamin A level is moderate, falling in percentile 60. Vitamin A is essential for the immune response and is also involved in other defenses against infectious agents. Most people can increase their level of vitamin A by the consumption of 5,000 I.U./day of retinyl palmitate. Beta carotene can be converted to vitamin A, but in many individuals this conversion is slow and ineffectual. It is a good idea to have good levels of *both*.

* The lipid protection ratio (not shown) is excellent, falling in percentile 86. This results mainly from a vitamin E value falling in percentile 93 and a cholesterol level falling in percentile 86. This is very satisfactory protection.

Vitamin E Is Nature's Master Antioxidant

Oxidative destruction of subcellular membrane lipids has been implicated along with other types of intracellular oxidative damage in the normal aging process and in the pathophysiology of a number of chronic diseases. Complex antioxidant mechanisms exist to limit the effects of these reactions. Vitamin E quenches free radicals effectively in small amounts, and evidence of its usefulness as a curative and preventive agent is accumulating. Results of controlled long-term intervention trials should be available soon.

Vitamin E was discovered at the University of California, Berkeley, in 1922 by Herbert Evans and Katherine Bishop, who observed that its deficiency caused fetal resorption in the rat. An active substance was isolated from wheat germ oil in 1936, also at Berkeley, and named "tocopherol" from the Greek words *tokos* (childbirth) and *pherein* (to carry) plus the -ol suffix designating a phenol or alcohol.

Vitamin E is a group of substances, the tocopherols and tocotrienols, found mainly in vegetable oils. Each has a chromanol head group and a phytyl side chain. The side chains of tocopherols are saturated, while those of tocotrienols contain three double bonds. Different numbers and placements of methyl groups in the aromatic ring produce α, β, γ, and δ forms of tocopherols and tocotrienols. Each form occurs in nature as a single stereoisomer. Synthetic vitamin E contains up to eight isomers, each with its own biological activity.

D-α-tocopherol is the most common type of vitamin E absorbed from the human diet, except that tocotrienols predominate in areas of the world where tropical plant oils are used for cooking and as sources of food. D-α-tocopherol is about 36 percent more active than the synthetic, isomeric mixture.

The function of vitamin E was disputed for decades and is not yet completely understood. An antioxidant property was evident once the chemical structure had been determined, for it resides in the phenolic hydroxyl group at C-6 on the aromatic ring. Readily oxidized, the tocopherols protect less susceptible compounds. Peroxidation of polyunsaturated fatty acids causes fats

Reprinted with permission from *Scientific American* magazine, *Science and Medicine* (March/April 1994): 54–63.

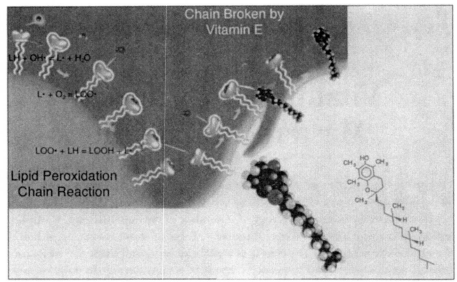

LH + OH· = L· + H₂O

L· + O₂ = LOO·

LOO· + LH = LOOH + L·

Lipid Peroxidation
Chain Reaction

Chain Broken by
Vitamin E

MARTIN BOSO

The α-tocopherol molecule

and oils to become rancid when exposed to air, and an early commercial use of vitamin E was to retard food spoilage. Biochemists supporting the view that the general antioxidant property was the key biologic activity could not show that lipid peroxidation occurred in animals, while those who favored a specific metabolic function were not able to identify one.

In the meantime, while the puzzling consequences of experimental vitamin E deficiency in animals were investigated, a barrage of unsubstantiated claims arose. With a kind of reverse logic, it has been argued that if a deficiency of vitamin E in animals causes lack of potency, then an excess in humans must cure impotence and act as an aphrodisiac. If a deficiency in animals causes muscle weakness and inability to tolerate exercise, then an excess in humans must lead to enhanced physical performance. Vitamin E is still promoted as a nostrum for ailments from cancer to arthritis. To skeptics it sounds like a twentieth-century version of the old snake oil remedy, but every faith has its believers, and vitamin E is being taken in large amounts by many people.

They may be right. Of itself, the variety of disease states induced in animals by vitamin E deficiency was an argument for a general rather than a specific function of the vitamin. Experiments by Al L. Tappel and colleagues at the University of California, Davis, beginning in the late 1950s directly demonstrated in vivo lipid peroxidation and the inhibitory effect of vitamin E. By blocking oxidation of lipids in subcellular membranes, vitamin E may have a role in defending the body against diseases. Quite small amounts of vitamin E are protective; much larger amounts taken as dietary supplements are unlikely to be harmful and may be beneficial.

Vitamin E Neutralizes Free Radicals

During normal energy metabolism, electrons are passed from foodstuffs down the electron transport chain in mitochondria to oxygen molecules, which accept electrons and protons to form water. The cell harnesses the energy released as ATP. But there are "leaks" in the electron transport chain, points at which single electrons can escape to transform atoms or molecules into free radicals. For example, a superoxide radical is formed when molecular oxygen accepts a single electron.

Superoxide, like other free radicals, is highly reactive, and one reaction in which it can engage is dismutation, to form hydrogen peroxide. Hydroxide ions and reactive hydroxyl radicals are formed from hydrogen peroxide in the presence of metal ions. Superoxide radicals, hydroxyl radicals, and hydrogen peroxide are the so-called excited oxygen or reactive oxygen species, and they cause intracellular oxidative damage in several ways. By reacting with DNA, for example, free radicals can induce mutagenic alterations.

Polyunsaturated fatty acids, susceptible to oxidative chain reactions at their double bonds, are present in plasma membranes and in mitochondrial membrane glycerophospholipids. Free radical lipid peroxidation propagates through polyunsaturated fatty acids, each completed peroxidation producing one of a variety of products and a new fatty acid peroxyl radical. In theory, oxidation of a single membrane lipid molecule by a single hydroxyl radical could start a chain reaction that would destroy the entire membrane.

Antioxidant mechanisms have evolved to stop the oxidative processes. Some antioxidants are enzymes that destroy superoxide radicals (superoxide dismutase) and peroxides (peroxidases and catalase). Others are molecules such as ferritin that bind tightly to metal ions and prevent the breakdown of hydrogen peroxide. Vitamin E interrupts the chain of membrane lipid peroxidation and is thus a "chain-breaking" antioxidant. The reaction of a lipid peroxyl radical with a vitamin E molecule interrupts peroxidation by producing a hydroperoxide and a vitamin E radical, both of which are relatively unreactive.

The vitamin E radical, or chromanoxyl radical, can follow one of several pathways. If it reacts with another chromanoxyl radical, with an alkoxyl radical, or with a peroxyl radical, the result is unreactive products with no further free radical scavenging activity. Alternatively, it can be reduced back to a functional vitamin E molecule.

Though it is the major, if not the only, chain-breaking antioxidant in mitochondrial membranes, vitamin E is present at extremely low concentrations,

Assays and Units

The earliest method of testing for the activity of vitamin E was a rat fetal resorption assay. Vitamin E–depleted female rats impregnated by normal males were kept on diets containing various amounts of the substance being assayed. The International Unit of vitamin E activity was based on the amount of vitamin E needed to prevent fetal resorption.

Other assay methods, equally tedious and insensitive, measured the ability of vitamin E to prevent deficiency symptoms in animals. Chromatography and sensitive electrochemical methods now allow direct measurement of the vitamin E content of a sample with ease. High-performance liquid chromatography enables detection of the presence of any form of tocopherol or tocotrienol in a sample, down to the pico-mole level, in fifteen minutes. Being able to record the exact amounts of compounds in a mixture rather than using the vague term "vitamin E activity" has clear advantages.

The contrast between the two kinds of assay procedures, one based on the appearance of deficiency symptoms and the other on chemical composition, raises a larger question about vitamin E. If its function depends only on its presence, then bioassays are useful and International Units are handy, but if its effects vary according to the specific tocopherol or tocotrienol content, then more sophisticated assays and more precise units of measurement are required.

Fairly early in the history of vitamin E research, it was clear that the antioxidant effects of the four tocopherols were different ($\alpha > \beta > \gamma > \delta$). Work in our laboratory with in vitro membrane systems has shown that the most common of the tocotrienols, D-α-tocotrienol, has forty to sixty times the antioxidant potency of D-α-tocopherol. While such differences have yet to be demonstrated in animals, they point to the necessity for careful discrimination among the various forms of vitamin E. Most research uses D-α-tocopherol, which is the most common naturally occurring form.

Each tocopherol and tocotrienol has its own conversion rate between mg and I.U. As a rough rule of thumb, 1 mg of natural "vitamin E" is equivalent to 1.5 I.U. of D-α-tocopherol, and 1 mg of synthetic vitamin E is equivalent to 1 I.U. of D,L-α-tocopherol.

usually less than 0.1 nmol per milligram of membrane protein or, in other words, one molecule per 1,000 to 2,000 membrane phospholipid molecules. Lipid peroxyl radicals can be generated in membranes at the rate of 1 to 5 nmol per milligram of membrane protein per minute, yet destructive oxidation of membrane lipids does not normally occur, nor is vitamin E rapidly depleted.

There must be an extremely efficient mechanism for regenerating or recycling vitamin E in order to sustain such minute but effective concentrations. Recycling of vitamin E by both enzymatic and nonenzymatic pathways has been demonstrated by us in artificial membrane systems, in microsomes, and in mitochondria.

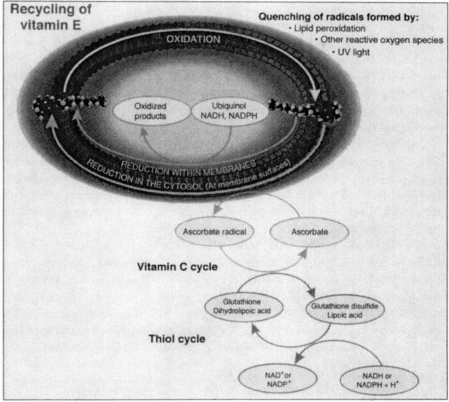

MARTIN BOSO

Chromanoxyl radicals are reduced to "native" vitamin E molecules in a complex and highly efficient system involving ubiquinol (coenzyme Q), vitamin C, and glutathione. Elements of the hypothetical mechanism have been worked out in model systems; confirmation of the theoretical and experimental biochemistry in an intact organism still lies ahead.

Deficiency States Are Unusual

Besides fetal resorption in the rat, a necrotizing myopathy of both skeletal and cardiac muscle in several animal species results from a deficiency of vitamin E. In immature animals of some of those species, adequate dietary vitamin E does not by itself reverse the myopathy; there must be adequate selenium as well. Other deficiency diseases, such as a liver necrosis in pigs, rats, and mice, are reversible by either vitamin E or selenium.

Probably because biologically active vitamin E is continually being recycled and not consumed, clinical signs of its deficiency cannot be induced in human adults. In an early experiment conducted by Max Horwitt at the Elgin State Hospital, volunteers were kept on diets containing no more than 4 milligrams of tocopherol per day for up to five years without developing any clinical signs of vitamin E deficiency, although their erythrocytes showed less resistance to induced peroxidation and a decrease in survival time.

There is a form of spinocerebellar degeneration produced by low levels of vitamin E owing to chronic fat malabsorption. The disorder has been described in both adults and children, some of whom had plasma levels of vitamin E that were not detectable at all. Recognition of vitamin E deficiency and restoration of normal vitamin E status stabilize and may reverse the neurologic degeneration.

Children are born with relatively low tocopherol levels. Premature infants have even less vitamin E and transiently are not able to absorb it. The consequent absence of adequate protection against membrane lipid oxidation is presumably involved in the pathogenesis of hemolytic anemia in prematures, whose risk is increased by the administration of iron because of its role in oxidative processes.

The use of oxygen to alleviate respiratory distress in prematures accelerates oxidative reactions and is associated with bronchopulmonary dysplasia, retrolental fibroplasia, and intravascular cerebral hemorrhages. In fact, retrolental fibroplasia was the first human disease to be linked to low levels of vitamin E, in 1949. Supplemental vitamin E may be helpful when oxygen must be administered to premature infants. If used, it is given intramuscularly or in very high oral doses because it is poorly absorbed by the premature infant's gut.

Lipid Peroxidation Is Associated with Human Diseases

Oxidative processes are implicated in the pathophysiology of many diseases. Laboratory findings and population studies have established the associations, and interventions are being tried. The interlinked nature of antioxidant mechanisms makes it difficult to isolate the effects of vitamin E supplementation in most instances, but it should be possible to define an optimal daily requirement for vitamin E more accurately than has been done in the past.

Oxidative modification of polyunsaturated fatty acids, cholesterol, and apoprotein B in low-density lipoproteins degrades the lipoproteins, which are taken up by macrophages. The result is foam cells, and aggregations of foam cells are the fatty streaks on which atherosclerotic plaques develop. Protection

---

Oxidative membrane damage has been implicated in:

• Cardiovascular disease	• Immune system dysfunction
• Carcinogenesis	• Cataracts
• Neurologic disorders	• Arthritis

Assessment of Lipid Peroxidation in Vivo

Two common methods measure secondary products, and neither is perfect. The **thiobarbituric acid** reaction usually uses plasma, easy to sample and to store. Heated with the sample at low pH, TBA is assumed to react with malondialdehyde, resulting in a pink product whose absorbance at 532 nm is taken as an indication of lipid peroxidation.

Other aldehydes, and indeed other chemicals in plasma, react with TBA, and the heating itself accelerates lipid peroxidation and triggers decomposition of lipid peroxidation products. Unless carefully controlled, the TBA assay may give values that are tens or even hundreds of times higher than the actual values of MDA in plasma. Furthermore, how well plasma reflects whole-body lipid peroxidation is not clear, nor is it known what components of plasma may be oxidized.

Hydrocarbon gases produced by lipid peroxidation are the basis for the measurement of **breath pentane.** Noninvasive and capable of being continuously monitored, the breath pentane assay is cumbersome and complicated, and its use is more or less restricted to research applications. The assumption is that increased lipid peroxidation results in increased pentane production and that the gas must ultimately be released in the lungs. Exhaled air can be collected, condensed, and stored in liquid nitrogen, and assayed for hydrocarbons by HPLC.

Hydrocarbon gases are also produced by gastrointestinal bacteria and are components of air pollution. The rate of metabolism, the iron content of various tissues, the antioxidant intake, and the metabolic conversion of pentane to pentanol all complicate the assay.

of low-density lipoproteins against oxidation has been observed in cell cultures containing various concentrations of vitamin E. In animal studies as well, vitamin E has been shown to have a protective effect and possibly to reverse established atherosclerotic lesions.

As part of an epidemiologic investigation, the WHO/MONICA study, ischemic heart disease mortality was correlated with risk factors across a number of European populations. The strongest link was between decreased mortality and high plasma concentrations of vitamins E and A, attributed to greater amounts of green and yellow vegetables in southern European diets. Reports from this large survey triggered interest in the "Mediterranean" or "vegetarian-type" diet now being widely touted.

An added benefit obtained from supplemental vitamin E has been suggested by reported findings from the Nurses' Health Study, in which 87,000 healthy women were followed for eight years. Those who took 100 mg or more of vitamin E per day had 36 percent less chance of developing heart diseases than those who did not, and if supplements were taken for more than two years, the risk dropped by more than 40 percent.

To consider a clinical situation, the major tissue damage seen in ischemia-reperfusion injury occurs not during ischemia but during reperfu-

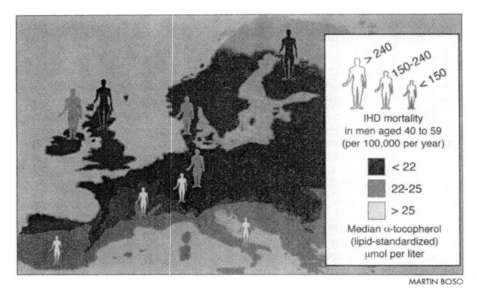

IHD mortality
in men aged 40 to 59
(per 100,000 per year)

< 22

22-25

> 25

Median α-tocopherol
(lipid-standardized)
μmol per liter

MARTIN BOSO

Blood levels of vitamin E were inversely correlated with mortality from ischemic heart disease in a cross-cultural survey of European populations. The data were reported by Fred Gey of the University of Bern.

sion. When deoxygenated blood is used for reperfusion, there is less tissue damage. Although the mechanism is debated, there is agreement that reactive oxygen species generated during reperfusion cause most of the damage. Hence vitamin E and other antioxidants should reduce ischemia-reperfusion injury.

In our laboratory, hearts from rats fed a diet supplemented with vitamin E experienced 70 percent better recovery on reperfusion as measured by enzyme release from damaged cardiac muscle after mechanical recovery. Others have reported similar results, and in some hospitals it is now routine to add antioxidants to the bathing medium during open heart surgery.

Populations exposed to high levels of ultraviolet radiation have the highest incidence of cutaneous melanoma, and the incidence of this disease has doubled in the United States over the past decade. Recent work from our laboratory and others indicates that free radicals are involved in UV-induced skin cancer and that antioxidants can play a role in its prevention.

The hypothetical steps in UV-induced skin cancer are (1) ultraviolet light induces the formation of free radicals in skin; (2) antioxidant defenses nullify free radicals, but if the dose of UV light is too great, the defenses will be overwhelmed; (3) the resulting free radical load causes damage to proteins, lipids, and DNA.

Using the hairless mouse as a model, we found decreased concentrations of all major antioxidants in the skin, and a simultaneous increase in lipid hydroperoxides, when the animals were irradiated with doses of ultraviolet light in the range commonly encountered by humans, equivalent to a few minutes to a few hours in the sun. Administering vitamin E before irradiation, as a dietary supplement or topically, reduced the level of UV-induced lipid hydroperoxide formation by two-thirds.

Studies by others, notably Homer Black, have shown that dietary supplementation with a combination of antioxidants including vitamin E reduced the incidence of skin tumors in irradiated mice and also that mice fed a diet high in polyunsaturated fats experienced more tumors than those fed diets lower in polyunsaturated fats. Mammary, colon, esophageal, and oral cancers have also been studied in laboratory animals, and vitamin E has been shown to be effective in reducing the incidence of tumors in the majority of studies.

As with atherosclerosis, epidemiologic studies suggest a possible role for antioxidants in cancer prevention. A case-control study of cancer patients in Finland found that those with low plasma vitamin E and selenium levels were at higher risk of dying than those with high antioxidant levels. American women with cervical dysplasia or cancer had lower levels of β-carotene and vitamin E than controls. Both Japanese and U.S. lung cancer patients had lower plasma vitamin E levels than matched controls.

No case-control study, however, can distinguish cause from effect. Among prospective studies in the United States, blood vitamin E levels were lower in subjects who subsequently developed lung cancer than in controls. A high intake of fiber, carotene, and vitamins C and E was associated with a lower risk of oral and pharyngeal cancer in black American men. People who took vitamin E supplements were found to have a lower risk of developing oral and pharyngeal cancer than people who did not.

Overall, Gladys Block of the University of California, Berkeley, analyzed 130 studies of the relationship between dietary intake or blood levels of antioxidants, or both, and the subsequent development of a variety of different cancers. She found that in 120, increased levels of antioxidants were associated with decreased cancer risk.

Problems plague this area of investigation, besides that of separating out the influences of the various antioxidants. Measurements must be made soon after blood samples are drawn because vitamin E is unstable. The vitamin E content at the time the samples were taken cannot be reliably determined after years in cold storage, a difficulty that vitiates the results of numerous early studies and some more recent ones.

Evidence for a preventive or curative role may be scant, but supplemental vitamin E may be useful during cancer chemotherapy. Anticancer agents such

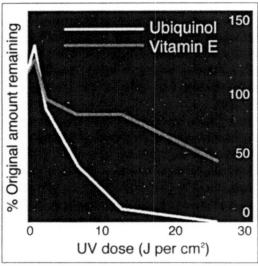

MARTIN BOSO

Defense of the skin against UV-induced cancer by antioxidants is suggested by animal experiments that showed steadily decreasing antioxidant concentrations and increasing amounts of lipid hydroperoxides with increasing exposure to UV light. Ubiquinol diminishes first, presumably because it is consumed by the reduction of vitamin E radicals.

as doxorubicin that generate reactive oxygen species damage normal tissue as well as cancerous tissue. Vitamin E and other antioxidants seem to protect healthy tissue from free radical attack while allowing chemotherapy to destroy cancer cells. Patients whose antioxidant status has been bolstered during chemotherapy seem to tolerate it better, increasing the likelihood that they will complete the course of treatment.

Antioxidants May Improve Performance and Extend Life Span

Oxygen consumption by working muscles can increase by a hundred times or more during exercise. Wherever there is more oxygen, there are more free radicals, so that damage to cells induced by reactive oxygen species should also increase during strenuous exercise. Kelvin Davies, formerly at Berkeley and now at Albany Medical College, demonstrated free radical formation and lipid peroxidation in the muscles of strenuously exercised animals.

With training, there is a concomitant increase in antioxidant defenses. However, Eric Witt, of our group at Berkeley, has shown that even highly trained college oarsmen have increased plasma lipid peroxidation after a strenuous exercise bout. Untrained rats develop not only signs of lipid peroxidation but also oxidative protein damage in their muscles when they are exercised strenuously. Vitamin E can significantly reduce the damage.

Carefully controlled studies by Witt and others failed to support exaggerated claims that antioxidants improve physical performance, with one exception. Mountain climbers given 400 I.U. of vitamin E per day showed improved physical performance and decreased breath pentane output during prolonged exposure to high altitudes, in a study done by Irene Simon-Schnass.

There is a remarkably consistent inverse correlation between metabolic rate and life span: the faster an organism uses oxygen, the more quickly it seems to age. Thus the constant appearance of free radicals during normal energy metabolism may be an important and even overriding factor in aging. If this is so, then antioxidant supplementation should slow the aging process. In animal experiments, average life span has been increased by supplementing diets with a variety of antioxidants, increases of 10 percent to 30 percent being reported. But such supplementation does not generally extend maximum life span.

Studies of aging human subjects show that vitamin E and other antioxidants can reverse some of the events of aging to some extent. For example, cell-mediated immunity tends to decline with age. In a study of subjects over 60, supplementation with vitamin E improved delayed-type hypersensitivity. In Poland, blood lipid peroxide levels were evaluated in people aged 60 to 100 who were then asked to take antioxidant supplements for a year. Those receiving vitamin E experienced a 26 percent decrease in lipid peroxides over the course of the study.

Daily Requirements Vary with Diet

The National Research Council first established Recommended Daily Allowances (RDAs) for vitamins in 1948, based on the prevention of observable deficiency syndromes. Vitamin E was omitted at first because of the difficulty of inducing clinical deficiency states. An RDA of 30 I.U. was established more or less arbitrarily in 1968. It was reduced in 1974 to 15 I.U. for men and 12 for women, since redefined as 10 tocopherol equivalents (10 mg of D-α-tocopherol) for men and 8 tocopherol equivalents for women.

Taking the antioxidant property of vitamin E as paramount, it is clear that the daily requirement depends on the individual diet. Someone who consumes a diet high in polyunsaturated fat, more susceptible to peroxidation, would benefit more from a high vitamin E intake. Dietary habits being what they are, such a person's sources of vitamin E are likely to be vegetable oils used in food processing.

At the high end of the scale, vitamin E causes few side effects in animals even at massive dosage levels, and those effects are minor and reversible. Mice

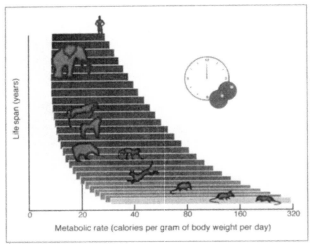

Possible aging effects of energy metabolism emerge when energy consumption is plotted against life span. The diagram is adapted from one originally prepared by Richard G. Cutler of the Gerontology Research Center, National Institute on Aging.

MARTIN BOSO

have been given single doses roughly the equivalent of a human adult taking 3,500,000 I.U. without adverse effects. Doses up to the equivalent of 5,000 I.U. per day for 10 to 60 days caused only a possible increase in coagulation time because of interference with vitamin K metabolism. Amounts equivalent to about 200,000 I.U. per day for two to three months resulted in increased liver weight, decreased hematocrit and hemoglobin, interstitial inflammation, and adenomatous pulmonary hyperplasia; these effects were not seen at doses up to an equivalent of 50,000 I.U. per day.

Unsubstantiated claims for the therapeutic effectiveness of vitamin E some years ago were accompanied by equally exaggerated notions of its side effects, notably dizziness, giddiness, intestinal cramps, and emotional disturbances. The supposed side effects disappeared along with many of the putative benefits when placebo-controlled, double-blind studies were done.

The World Health Organization considers daily doses of vitamin E up to 150 milligrams to be "absolutely safe" and doses between 150 and 720 milligrams to be a "range without side effects." From 720 milligrams to 3,000 milligrams, transient gastrointestinal complaints begin to appear along with increased coagulation time, which is a problem in patients with vitamin K deficiency or who are taking anticoagulants. Studies of doses above 3,000 milligrams per day have not been done in humans. Topical preparations containing synthetic α-tocopherol may cause skin irritation, while those containing α-tocopherol acetate do not.

The average American consumes 11 to 13 I.U. of α-tocopherol per day and much smaller amounts of the less common tocopherols and tocotrienols. Depending on the individual diet, the range is probably from 5 I.U. or less up to 30 I.U. or more. On the average intake, the average blood level is about 23 μmol per liter. A widely promoted multivitamin supplement provides 30 I.U. per day, which is almost certainly safe and which may be beneficial.

Biokinetics and Regulatory Functions Are Being Studied

The biokinetics and tissue absorption of vitamin E have not been well studied in humans. Dietary vitamin E is absorbed with fat and transported in chylomicrons to the liver and other tissues. There is an α-tocopherol-binding protein in the liver; there may be others for the other tocopherols and the tocotrienols. Tocopherols in plasma tend to be associated with phospholipid-rich lipoproteins, but tocotrienols are primarily found in triglyceride-rich lipoproteins. Therefore, different pathways must exist for the incorporation of these compounds into lipoproteins. Specificity is also expressed at the interfaces between plasma lipoproteins, probably including chylomicrons, and various tissues. Adipose tissue becomes enriched in tocotrienols, while in our research we have observed that most other tissues contain equivalent amounts of α-tocopherol and α-tocotrienol when equivalent amounts of both compounds are fed.

Antioxidants may exert regulatory effects on cellular signaling mecha-

Foods High in Vitamin E
(Amount needed to get 30 I.U.)

Wheat germ oil	1 tablespoon
Sunflower seeds	1½ ounces
Sunflower oil	3 tablespoons
Safflower oil	3½ tablespoons
Almonds	3 ounces
Peanut oil	8 tablespoons
Mayonnaise	11 tablespoons
Margarine (soft)	6 ounces
Wheat germ	6 ounces
Margarine (stick)	7 ounces
Peanuts (dry roasted)	10 ounces
Peanut butter	12 ounces
Soybean oil	13 tablespoons
Butter	2 pounds
Brown rice (boiled)	2¼ pounds
Asparagus	2½ pounds
Spinach	2½ pounds
Broiled liver	7 pounds
Baked shrimp	7½ pounds
Whole wheat bread	124 slices
Peas	8 pounds
Broccoli	9½ pounds
Eggs	8 dozen
Bacon	10 pounds

Sources of Vitamin E in the American Diet
(USDA Nationwide Food Consumption Survey, 1987–88)

Margarine	13%
Mayonnaise	10%
Fortified breakfast cereal	6%
Shortening	5%
Salad dressing	3%
Peanut butter	3%
Eggs	2%
Soybean oil	2%
Potato chips	2%
Milk	2%
Tomato sauce	1%
Apples	1%
All other sources	51%

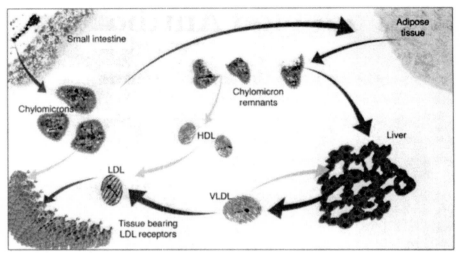

MARTIN BOSO

Transport of α**-tocopherol** from intestines to tissues may involve three pathways: hepatic secretion of VLDL that is delipidated to LDL; transfer via HDL and LDL to tissues with LDL receptors; and direct release upon catabolism of chylomicrons by circulating lipoprotein lipase.

nisms, including gene expression. A nuclear transcription factor, NFκB, present in many cells that activates and down-regulates genetic systems, including viral proliferation, has been shown to be activated by reactive oxygen species. Tumor necrosis factor and phorbol esters activate NFκB in human T-cells. Thiol antioxidants such as N-acetylcysteine and α-lipoic acid are potent inhibitors of NFκB activation. Recent studies in our laboratory have demonstrated that α-tocopherol succinate and α-tocopherol acetate may inhibit NFκB activation by tumor necrosis factor and phorbol esters.

Influences on the cyclooxygenase and lipooxygenase pathways of arachidonic acid metabolism have also been suggested.

Classically, a vitamin is defined as a substance necessary in small amounts in the diet to assist normal metabolism and whose lack causes one or several clearly defined deficiency states. Vitamin E has not appeared to fit the classical definition because the conditions that it prevents take years to develop. This view has been supported by epidemiological and laboratory studies. Clinical trials now in progress will redefine vitamin E requirements in terms of a dosage necessary for optimal functioning. Continuing laboratory efforts are certain to enlarge understanding of the intricately related antioxidant mechanisms that function in living cells and may at last establish with certainty the biologic functions of vitamin E.

Notes

Recent Review

Packer, Lester, and Jürgen Fuchs, eds. October 1992. *Vitamin E in health and disease.* New York: Marcel Dekker.

Original Papers

Block, Gladys, et al. July–August 1992. Carcinogenesis. *Nutrition and Cancer* 18:1–29.

Gey, K. Fred, et al. January 1991. Vitamin E and ischemic heart disease in European populations. *Journal of Clinical Nutrition* 53:326S–34S.

Halliwell, Barry, and Susanna Chirico. April 1993. Significance of lipid peroxidation in human disease. *American Journal of Clinical Nutrition* 57:715S–25S.

Rimm, Eric B., et al. 20 May 1993. Coronary disease vs. vitamin E consumption in men. *New England Journal of Medicine* 328:1450–56.

Serbinova, Elena A., et al. 1991. Recycling. *Free Radicals in Biology and Medicine* 10:263–75.

Stampfer, Meir J., et al. 20 May 1993. Vitamin E consumption and the risk of coronary disease in women. *New England Journal of Medicine* 328:1444–49.

The books listed below are excellent sources of information on topics covered in *The Antioxidant Miracle.*

2   The Antioxidant Network in Action

Cadenas, E., and L. Packer, eds. 1996. *Antioxidants in health and disease.* In Vol. 3 of *Handbook of antioxidants,* edited by L. Packer and J. Fuchs. New York: Marcel Dekker.

3   Free Radicals: Both Enemy and Friend

Emerit, I., and B. Chance, eds. 1992. *Free radicals and aging.* Basel, Switzerland: Berkhäuser Verlag.

Halliwell, F., and J. M. C. Gutteridge, eds. October 1998. *Free radicals in biology and medicine.* 3d ed. Oxford, England: Clarendon Press.

Packer, L., ed. 1984. *Oxygen radicals in biological systems.* In *Methods in enzymology.* Vol. 105. Orlando, Fla.: Academic Press.

———. 1994. *Oxygen radicals in biological systems.* In *Methods in enzymology.* Vol. 233. San Diego: Academic Press.

———. 1994. *Oxygen radicals in biological systems.* In *Methods in enzymology.* Vol. 234. San Diego: Academic Press.

———. 1996. *Nitric oxide: Sources and detection of NO; NO synthase.* In *Methods in enzymology.* Vol. 268. San Diego: Academic Press.

———. 1996. *Nitric oxide: Physiological and pathological processes.* In *Methods in enzymology.* Vol. 269. San Diego: Academic Press.

———. 1998. *Oxidants and antioxidants.* In *Methods in enzymology.* Vol. 299. San Diego: Academic Press.

———. 1998. *Oxidants and antioxidants.* In *Methods in enzymology.* Vol. 300. San Diego: Academic Press.

———. 1998. *Nitrogen monoxide (NO).* In *Methods in enzymology.* Vol. 301. San Diego: Academic Press.

————, and A. N. Glazer, eds. 1990. *Oxygen radicals in biological systems. Oxidants and antioxidants.* In *Methods in enzymology.* Vol. 186. San Diego: Academic Press.

————, and A. Ong, eds. 1998. *Biological oxidants and antioxidants: Molecular mechanisms and health effects.* Champaign, Ill.: AOCS Press.

————, M. Hiramatsu, and T. Yoshikawa, eds. 1996. *Free radicals in brain physiology and disorders.* San Diego: Academic Press.

4   Lipoic Acid: The Universal Antioxidant

Fuchs, J., L. Packer, and G. Zimmer, eds. 1997. *Lipoic acid in health and disease.* In Vol. 6 of *Antioxidants in health and disease,* edited by L. Packer and J. Fuchs. New York: Marcel Dekker.

Packer, L., ed. 1995. *Biothiols: Monothiols and dithiols, protein thiols and thiyl radicals.* In *Methods in enzymology.* Vol. 251. San Diego: Academic Press.

————, and E. Cadenas, eds. 1995. *Biothiols in health and disease.* In Vol. 2 of *Antioxidants in health and disease,* edited by L. Packer and J. Fuchs. New York: Marcel Dekker.

5   Vitamin E: An Extraordinary Antioxidant

Krinsky, N. I., and H. Sies, eds. 1995. Antioxidant vitamins and β-carotene in disease prevention. *American Journal of Clinical Nutrition* 62, no. 6(S): 1299S–1540S.

Packer, L., and J. Fuchs, eds. 1993. *Vitamin E in health and disease.* Vol. 28. New York: Marcel Dekker.

6   Vitamin C: The Hub of the Network

Krinsky, N. I., and H. Sies, eds. 1995. Antioxidant vitamins and β-carotene in disease prevention. *American Journal of Clinical Nutrition* 62, no. 6 (S):1299S–1540S.

Packer, L., and J. Fuchs, eds. 1991. *Vitamin C in health and disease.* Vol. 5. New York: Marcel Dekker.

7   Coenzyme Q10: The Heart-Healthy Antioxidant

Littarru, G. P., et al., eds. 1997. *Biomedical and clinical aspects of coenzyme Q. Molecular aspects of medicine.* Vol. 18 (suppl.). Oxford, England: Elsevier Science.

Sinatra, S. T. 1998. *The coenzyme Q10 phenomenon*. New Canaan, Conn.: Keats Publishing.

8 Glutathione: Nature's Master Antioxidant

Packer, L., ed. 1995. *Biothiols: Monothiols and dithiols, protein thiols and thiyl radicals*. In *Methods in enzymology*. Vol. 251. San Diego: Academic Press.

————. 1995. *Biothiols: Glutathione and thioredoxin—Thiols in signal transduction and gene regulation*. In *Methods in enzymology*. Vol. 252. San Diego: Academic Press.

————, and E. Cadenas, eds. 1995. *Biothiols in health and disease*. In Vol. 2 of *Antioxidants in health and disease*, edited by L. Packer and J. Fuchs. New York: Marcel Dekker.

9 The Flavonoids: The Healing Power of Plants

Rice-Evans, C., and L. Packer, eds. 1997. *Flavonoids in health and disease*. In Vol. 7 of *Antioxidants in health and disease*, edited by L. Packer and J. Fuchs. New York: Marcel Dekker.

10 The Controversial Carotenoids

Blomhoff, R., ed. 1994. *Vitamin A in health and disease*. In Vol. 1 of *Antioxidants in health and disease*, edited by L. Packer and J. Fuchs. New York: Marcel Dekker.

Krinsky, N. I., and H. Sies, eds. 1995. Antioxidant vitamins and β-carotene in disease prevention. *American Journal of Clinical Nutrition* 62, no. 6 (S): 1299S–1540S.

Packer, L., ed. 1990. *Retinoids. Molecular and metabolic aspects*. In *Methods in enzymology*. Vol. 189. San Diego: Academic Press.

————. 1990. *Retinoids. Cell differentiation and clinical applications*. In *Methods in enzymology*. Vol. 190. San Diego: Academic Press.

————. 1992. *Carotenoids: Chemistry, separation, quantitation and antioxidation*. In *Methods in enzymology*. Vol. 213. San Diego: Academic Press.

————. 1993. *Carotenoids: Metabolism, genetics and biosynthesis*. In *Methods in enzymology*. Vol. 214. San Diego: Academic Press.

11 The Selenium Surprise

Burk, R. F., ed. 1994. *Selenium in biology and human health*. New York: Springer-Verlag.

Combs, G. F., and S. B. Combs. 1986. *The role of selenium in nutrition.* Orlando, Fla.: Academic Press.

12 Fulfilling the Antioxidant Miracle: Achieving Optimal Health

Cadenas, E., and L. Packer, eds. 1996. *Handbook of antioxidants.* In Vol. 3 of *Antioxidants in health and disease,* edited by L. Packer and J. Fuchs. New York: Marcel Dekker.

Cooper, K. H. 1994. *The antioxidant revolution.* Nashville, Tenn.: Thomas Nelson.

Frei, B., ed. 1994. *Natural antioxidants in human health and disease.* San Diego: Academic Press.

Montagnier, L., R. Olivier, and C. Pasquier, eds. 1998. *Oxidative stress in cancer, AIDS and neurodegenerative diseases.* In Vol. 1 of *Oxidative stress and disease,* edited by L. Packer and E. Cadenas. New York: Marcel Dekker.

Packer, L., ed. 1984. *Oxygen radicals in biological systems.* In *Methods in enzymology.* Vol. 105. Orlando, Fla.: Academic Press.

———. 1994. *Oxygen radicals in biological systems.* In *Methods in enzymology.* Vol. 233. San Diego: Academic Press.

———. 1994. *Oxygen radicals in biological systems.* In *Methods in enzymology.* Vol. 234. San Diego: Academic Press.

———. 1996. *Nitric oxide: Sources and detection of NO; NO synthase.* In *Methods in enzymology.* Vol. 268. San Diego: Academic Press.

———. 1996. *Nitric oxide: Physiological and pathological processes.* In *Methods in enzymology.* Vol. 269. San Diego: Academic Press.

———. On press. *Oxidants and antioxidants.* In *Methods in enzymology.* Vol. 299. San Diego: Academic Press.

———. On press. *Oxidants and antioxidants.* In *Methods in enzymology.* Vol. 300. San Diego: Academic Press.

———. On press. *Nitrogen monoxide (NO).* In *Methods in enzymology.* Vol. 301. San Diego: Academic Press.

———, and A. N. Glazer, eds. 1990. *Oxygen radicals in biological systems. Oxidants and antioxidants.* In *Methods in enzymology.* Vol. 186. San Diego: Academic Press.

———, and A. Ong, eds. 1998. *Biological oxidants and antioxidants: Molecular mechanisms and health effects.* Champaign, Ill.: AOCS Press.

———, M. Traber, and W. Xin, eds. 1996. *Proceedings of the International Symposium on Natural Antioxidants: Molecular mechanisms and health effects.* Champaign, Ill.: AOCS Press.

————, T. Yoshikawa, and M. Hiramatsu, eds. On press. *Antioxidant food supplements in human health*. San Diego: Academic Press.

Sen, C. K., L. Packer, and O. Hanninen, eds. 1994. *Exercise and oxygen toxicity*. Amsterdam: Elsevier.

Sies, H., ed. 1991. *Oxidative stress: Oxidants and antioxidants*. San Diego: Academic Press.

13   An Antioxidant Feast: Food Is Powerful Medicine

Madhavi, D. L., S. S. Deshpande, and D. K. Salunkhe, eds. 1996. *Food antioxidants: Technological, toxicological and health perspectives*. New York: Marcel Dekker.

Micozzi, M. S., and T. E. Moon, eds. 1992. *Macronutrients*. New York: Marcel Dekker.

Ohigashi, H., T. Osawa, J. Terao, S. Watanabe, and T. Yoshikawa, eds. 1997. *Food factors for chemistry and cancer prevention*. Tokyo: Springer-Verlag.

Pappas, A., ed. 1998. *Antioxidant status, diet, nutrition, and health*. Boca Raton, Fla.: CRC Press.

15   The Packer Plan: Antioxidants for Healthy, Beautiful Skin

Balin, A. K., and A. M. Kligman. 1989. *Aging and the skin*. New York: Raven Press.

Fuchs, J. 1992. *Oxidative injury in dermatopathology*. Berlin: Springer-Verlag.

1   The Antioxidant Miracle

Halliwell, B. 1996. Antioxidants in human health and disease. *Annual Review of Nutrition* 16:33–50.

———. 1994. Antioxidants: Sense or speculation? *Nutrition Today* 29:15–19.

Packer, L. 1993. Health effects of nutritional antioxidants [letter]: *Free Radical Biology and Medicine* 15:685–86.

2   The Antioxidant Network in Action

Packer, L. 1994. Vitamin E is nature's master antioxidant. *Scientific American: Science and Medicine* 1:54–63. (cf. Appendix.)

3   Free Radicals: Both Enemy and Friend

Angier, N. 1993. Free radicals: The price we pay for breathing. *New York Times Magazine*, 25 April.

Beckman, K. B., and B. N. Ames. 1998. The free radical theory of aging matures. *Physiological Reviews* 78 (2):547–81.

Church, D. F., and W. A. Pryor. 1985. Free-radical chemistry of cigarette smoke and its toxicological implications. *Environmental Health Prospectives* 64:111–26.

Finkel, T. 1998. Oxygen radicals and signaling. *Current Opinion in Cell Biology* 10 (2):248–53.

Harman, D. 1956. Aging: A theory based on free radical and radiation chemistry. *Journal of Gerontology* 11:298–300.

———. 1992. Free radical theory of aging: History. In *Free Radicals and Aging*, edited by I. Emerit and B. Chance. Basel, Switzerland: Berkhäuser Verlag.

Nakamura, H., K. Nakamura, and J. Yodoi. 1997. Redox regulation of cellular activation. *Annual Review of Immunology* 15:351–69.

Palmer, H. J., and K. E. Paulson. 1997. Reactive oxygen species and antioxidants in signal transduction and gene expression. *Nutrition Reviews* 55:353–61.

Pryor, W. A. 1991. The antioxidant nutrients and disease prevention—what do we know and what do we need to find out? *American Journal of Clinical Nutrition* 53 (suppl. 1):391–93.

Sen, C. K., and L. Packer. 1996. Antioxidant and redox regulation of gene transcription. *The Federation of American Societies for Experimental Biology (FASEB) Journal* 10 (7):709–20.

4   Lipoic Acid: The Universal Antioxidant

Bustamante, J., J. K. Lodge, L. Marcocci, H. J.Tritschler, L. Packer, and B. H. Rihn. 1998. a-lipoic acid in liver metabolism and disease. *Free Radical Biology & Medicine* 24:1023–39.

Kagan, V. E., E. A. Serbinova, T. Forte, G. Scita, and L. Packer. 1992. Recycling of vitamin E in human low density lipoproteins. *Journal of Lipid Research* 33:385–97.

———, A. Shvedova, E. Serbinova, S. Khan, C. Swanson, R. Powell, and L. Packer. 1992. Dihydrolipoic acid—a universal antioxidant both in the membrane and in the aqueous phase. *Biochemical Pharmacology* 44:1637–49.

Kilic, F., G. J. Handelman, E. Serbinova, L. Packer, and J. R. Trevithick. 1995. Modelling cortical cataractogenesis 17: In vitro effect of a-lipoic acid on glucose-induced lens membrane damage, a model of diabetic catarctogenesis. *Biochemistry and Molecular Biology International* 37:361–70.

Maitra, I., E. Serbinova, H. J. Tritschler, and L. Packer. 1995. Alpha-lipoic acid prevents buthionine sulfoximine-induced cataract formation in newborn rats. *Free Radical Biology & Medicine* 18:823–29.

Packer, L. 1996. Antioxidant defenses in biological systems: An overview. In *Proceedings of the International Symposium on Natural Antioxidants: Molecular Mechanisms and Health Effects,* edited by L. Packer, M. Traber, and W. Xin. Champaign, Ill.: AOCS Press.

———. 1996. Prevention of free radical damage in the brain—protection by alpha-lipoic acid. In *Free Radicals in Brain Physiology and Disorders,* edited by L. Packer, M. Hiramatsu, and T. Yoshikawa. San Diego: Academic Press.

———, and H. J. Tritschler. 1996. Alpha-lipoic acid—the metabolic antioxidant. *Free Radical Biology & Medicine* 20:625–26.

———, E. H. Witt, and H. J. Tritschler. 1995. Alpha-lipoic acid as a biological antioxidant. *Free Radical Biology & Medicine* 19:227–50.

———, E. H. Witt, and H. J. Tritschler. 1996. Antioxidant properties and clinical implications of alpha-lipoic acid and dihydrolipoic acid. *Handbook of Antioxidants,* edited by E. Cadenas and L. Packer. New York: Marcel Dekker.

———, H. J. Tritschler, and K. Wessel. 1997. Neuroprotection by the metabolic antioxidant a-lipoic acid. *Free Radical Biology & Medicine* 22 (1–2):359–78.

Panigrahi, M., Y. Sadguna, B. R. Shivakumar, S. Kolluri, S. Roy, L. Packer, and V. Ravindranath. 1996. Alpha-lipoic acid protects against reperfusion injury following cerebral ischemia in rats. *Brain Research* 717:184–88.

Sen, C. K., S. Roy, D. Han, and L. Packer. 1997. Regulation of cellular thiols in human lymphocytes by a∂-lipoic acid: A flow cytometric analysis. *Free Radical Biology & Medicine* 22:1241–57.

Sen, C., S. Roy, and L. Packer. 1997. Therapeutic potential of the antioxidant and redox properties of a-lipoic acid. In *Oxidative stress in cancer, AIDS, and neurodegenerative diseases,* edited by L. Montagnier, R. Olivier, and C. Pasquier. New York: Marcel Dekker.

Serbinova, E., S. Khwaja, A. Z. Reznick, and L. Packer. 1992. Thioctic acid protects against ischemia-reperfusion injury in the isolated perfused Langendorff heart. *Free Radical Research Communications* 17:49–58.

Suzuki, Y. J., M. Tsuchiya, and L. Packer. 1991. Thioctic acid and dihydrolipoic acid are novel antioxidants which interact with reactive oxygen species. Published erratum appears in *Free Radical Research Communications* 17 (2)(1992):155. *Free Radical Research Communications* 15:255–63.

Ziegler, D., and F. A. Gries. 1997. Alpha-lipoic acid in the treatment of diabetic peripheral and cardiac autonomic neuropathy. *Diabetes* 46 (suppl. 2):62–66.

5   Vitamin E: An Extraordinary Antioxidant

Bierenbaum, M. L., T. R. Watkins, A. Gapor, M. Geller, and A. C. Tomeo. 1995. Antioxidant effects of tocotrienols in patients with hyperlipidemia and carotid stenosis. *Lipids* 30:1179–83.

Brown, A. J. 1996. Acute effects of smoking cessation on antioxidant status. *Experimental Journal of Nutritional Biochemistry* 7:29–39.

Carroll, K. K., A. F. Chambers, A. Gapor, and N. Guthrie. 1997. Inhibition of proliferation of estrogen-receptor-negative MDA-MB-435 and -positive MCF-7 human breast cancer cells by palm tocotrienols and Tamoxifen, alone and in combination. *Journal of Nutrition* 127:544S–48S.

Christen, S., A. A. Woodall, M. K. Shigenaga, P. T. Southwell-Keely, M. W. Duncan, and B. N. Ames. 1997. g-tocopherol traps mutagenic electrophiles such as NOX and complements a-tocopherol: Physiological implications. *Proceedings of the National Academy of Sciences* 94:3217–22.

Cooney, R. V., A. A. Franke, P. J. Harwood, V. Hatch-Pigott, L. J. Custer, and L. Mordan. 1993. g-tocopherol detoxification of nitrogen dioxide: Superiority to a-tocopherol. *Proceedings of the National Academy of Sciences* 90:1771–75.

Diplock, A., L. Machlin, L. Packer, and W. A. Pryor., eds. 1989. Vitamin E: Biochemistry and health implications. *Annals of the New York Academy of Sciences.* Vol. 570.

Edmonds, S. E., P. G. Winyard, R. Guo, B. Kidd, P. Merry, A. Langrish-Smith, C. Hansen, S. Ramm, and D. R. Blake. 1997. Putative analgesic activity of repeated oral doses of vitamin E in the treatment of rheumatoid arthritis. Results of a prospective placebo-controlled double-blind trial. *Annals of the Rheumatic Diseases* 56 (11):649–55.

Elson, C. E., 1995. Suppression of mevalonate pathway indices by dietary isoprenoids: protective roles in cancer and cardiovascular disease. *Journal of Nutrition* 125:1666S–72S.

Esterbauer, H., J. Gebicki, H. Puhl, and G. Jurgens. 1992. The role of lipid peroxidation and antioxidants in oxidative modification of LDL. *Free Radical Biology & Medicine* 13 (4):341–90.

Goh, S. H., N. F. Hew, A. W. Norhanom, and M. Yadav. 1994. Inhibition of tumour promotion by various palm-oil tocotrienols. *International Journal of Cancer* 57:529–31.

Gohil, K., L. Rothfuss, J. Lang, and L. Packer. 1987. Effect of exercise training on tissue vitamin E and ubiquinone content. *Journal of Applied Physiology* 63 (4):1638–41.

Gould, M. N., J. D. Haag, W. S. Kennan, M. A. Tanner, and C. E. Elson. 1991. A comparison of tocopherol and tocotrienol for the chemoprevention of chemically induced rat mammary tumors. *American Journal of Clinical Nutrition* 53:1068S–70S.

Guthrie, N., A. Gapor, A. F. Chambers, and K. K. Carroll. 1997. Palm oil tocotrienols and plant flavonoids act with each other and with Tamoxifen in inhibiting proliferation and growth of estrogen receptor–negative MDA-MB-435 and -positive MCF-7 human breast cancer cells in culture. *Asia Pacific Journal of Clinical Nutrition* 6:41–45.

Henderson, B. E., L. N. Kolonel, R. Dworsky, D. Kerford, E. Mori, K. Singh, and H. Thevenot. 1986. Cancer incidence in the islands of the Pacific. *National Cancer Institute Monograph* 69:73–81.

Hirahara, F. 1987. Effects of d-a-tocopherol, d-g-tocopherol and d-a-tocotrienol on atherogenic diet fed rats after high-dose administration. *Nutr Rep Int* 36:161–67.

Khor, H. T., D. Y. Chieng, and K. K. Ong. 1995. Tocotrienols inhibit liver HMG-CoA reductase activity in the guinea pig. *Nutrition Research* 15:537–44.

Knekt, P. 1997. Vitamin E and cancer prevention: Methodological aspects of human studies. In *Food Factors for Chemistry and Cancer Prevention,* edited by H. Ohigashi, T. Osawa, J. Terao, S. Watanabe, and T. Yoshikawa. Tokyo: Springer-Verlag.

Kolonel, L. N., L. Marchand, J. H. Hankin, F. Bach, L. Wilkins, M. Stacewicz, P. Bowen, L. S. Beecher, F. Lauden, P. Baques, R. Daniel, L. Serunatu, and B. Henderson. 1991. Relation of nutrient intakes and smoking in relation to cancer incidence in Cook Islanders. *Proceedings of the American Association for Cancer Research* 32:472.

Komiyama, K., K. Iuzuka, M. Yamaoka, H. Watanabe, N. Tsuchiya, and I. Umezawa. 1989. Studies on the biological activity of tocotrienols. *Chemical Pharmacology Bulletin* 37:1369–71.

Kooyenga, D. K., M. Geller, T. R. Watkins, A. Gapor, E. Diakoumakis, and M. L. Bierenbaum. 1997. Palm oil antioxidants: Effects in patients with hyperlipidemia and carotid stenosis—2-year experience. *Asia Pacific Journal of Clinical Nutrition* 6:72–75.

Leske, M. C., L. T. Chylack Jr., Q. He, S. Y. Wu, E. Schoenfeld, J. Friend, and J. Wolfe. 1998. Antioxidant vitamins and nuclear opacities: The longitudinal study of cataract. *Ophthalmology* 105 (5):831–36.

Meydani, M., W. J. Evans, G. Handelman, L. Biddle, R. A. Fielding, S. N. Meydani, J. Burrill, M. A. Fiatarone, J. B. Blumberg, and J. G. Cannon. 1993. Protective effect of vitamin E on exercise-induced oxidative damage in young and older adults. *American Journal of Physiology* 264 (5 pt. 2):R992–98.

Nesaretnam, K., N. Guthrie, A. F. Chambers, and K. K. Carol. 1995. Effect of tocotrienols on the growth of a human breast cancer cell line in culture. *Lipids* 30:1139–43.

Ngah, W. W., Z. Jarien, M. M. San, A. Marzuki, G. M. Top, N. A. Shamaan, and K. A. Kadir. 1991. Effect of tocotrienols on hepatocarcinogenesis induced by 2-acetylaminofluorene in rats. *American Journal of Clinical Nutrition* 53:1076S–81S.

Ohrvall, M., G. Sudlof, et al. 1996. Gamma-, but not alpha-tocopherol levels in serum are reduced in coronary heart disease patients. *Journal of Internal Medicine* 239:111–17.

Packer, L. 1984. Vitamin E, physical exercise and tissue damage in animals. *Medical Biology* 62:105–09.

———. 1991. Protective role of vitamin E in biological systems. *American Journal of Clinical Nutrition* 53 (suppl. 4):1050–55.

———. 1992. Interactions among antioxidants in health and disease: Vitamin E and its redox cycle. *Proceedings of the Society for Experimental Biology and Medicine* 200 (2):271–76.

———. 1997. Oxidants, antioxidant nutrients and the athlete. *Journal of Sports Science* 15:353–63.

———, and J. R. Smith. 1974. Extension of the lifespan of cultured normal human diploid cells by vitamin E. *Proceedings of the National Academy of Sciences* 71:4763–67.

———, and S. Landvik. 1990. Vitamin E in biological systems. *Advances in Experimental Medicine and Biology* 264:93–103.

———, and Y. Suzuki. 1993. Vitamin E and α-lipoate: Role in antioxidant recycling and activation of the NF-kB transcription factor. *Journal of Molecular Aspects of Medicine* 14:229–39.

———, A. Z. Reznick, I. Simon-Schnass, and S. V. Landvik. 1993. Significance of Vitamin E for the athlete. *Vitamin E in Health and Disease*, edited by J. Fuchs and L. Packer. New York: Marcel Dekker.

———, M. Podda, C. Weber, and M. G. Traber. 1996. Simultaneous determination of tissue tocopherols, tocotrienols, ubiquinols, and ubiquinones. *Journal of Lipid Research* 37:893–901.

Parker, R. A., B. C. Pearce, R. W. Clark, D. A. Gordon, and J. K. Wright. 1993. Tocotrienols regulate cholesterol production in mammalian cells by posttranscriptional suppression of 3-hydroxy-3-methylglutaryl coenzyme A reductase. *Journal of Biological Chemistry* 268:11230–38.

Pearce, B. C., R. A. Parker, M. E. Deason, A. A. Qureshi, and J. K. Wright. 1992. Hypocholesterolemic activity of synthetic and natural tocotrienols. *Journal of Medical Chemistry* 35:3595–606.

Pereira, O. M., J. R. Smith, and L. Packer. 1976. Photosensitization of human diploid cell cultures by intracellular flavins and protection by antioxidants. *Photochemistry and Photobiology* 24:237–42.

Qureshi, A. A.,W. C. Burger, C. E. Elson, and D. M. Peterson. 1986. The structure of an inhibitor of cholesterol biosynthesis isolated from barley. *Journal of Biological Chemistry* 261:10544–50.

———, B. A. Bradlow, W. A. Salser, and L. D. Brace. 1997. Novel tocotrienols of rice bran modulate cardiovascular disease risk parameters of hypercholesterolemic humans. *Nutritional Biochemistry* 8:290–98.

———, B. C. Pearce, R. M. Nor, A. Gapor, D. M. Peterson, and C. E. Elson. 1996. a-tocopherol attenuates the impact of a-tocotrienol in hepatic HMG-CoA reductase activity in chickens. *Journal of Nutrition* 126:389–94.

———, B. A. Bradlow, L. Brace, J. Manganello, D. M. Peterson, B. C. Pearce, J. J. K. Wright, A. Gapor, and C. E. Elson. 1995. Response of hypercholesterolemic subjects to administration of tocotrienols. *Lipids* 30:1171–77.

———, N. Qureshi, J. O. Haslaer-Rapaez, F. E. Weber, V. Chaudhary, T. D. Crenshaw, A. Gapor, A. Ong, Y. H. Chong, D. Peterson, and J. Rapaez. 1991. Dietary tocotrienols reduce concentrations of plasma cholesterol, apoB, thromboxane B2, and platelet factor 4 in pigs with inherited hyperlipidemias. *American Journal of Clinical Nutrition* 53:1042S–46S.

Regnström, J., J. Nilsson, P. Moldeus, K. Ström, P. Bavenholm, P. Tornvall, and A. Hamsten. 1996. Inverse relation between the concentration of low-density-lipoprotein vitamin E and severity of coronary artery disease. *American Journal of Clinical Nutrition* 63 (3):377–85.

Rimm, E. B., M. J. Stampfer, A. Ascherio, E. Giovannucci, G. A. Colditz, and W. C. Willett. 1993. Vitamin E consumption and the risk of coronary heart disease in men. *New England Journal of Medicine* 328 (20):1450–56.

Rosen, P., and L. Packer. 1997. Vitamin E and diabetes mellitus. *Diabetes und Stoffwechsel* 6:2–3.

Serbinova, E., V. Kagan, D. Han, and L. Packer. 1991. Free radical recycling and intramembrane mobility in the antioxidant properties of alpha-tocopherol and alpha-tocotrienol. *Free Radical Biology & Medicine* 10:263–75.

———, and S. Khwaja. 1992. Palm oil vitamin E protects against ischemia/reperfusion injury in the isolated perfused Langendorff heart. *Nutrition Research* 12 (suppl. 1):203–13.

Stampfer, M. J., C. H. Hennekens, J. E. Manson, G. A. Colditz, B. Rosner, and W. C. Willett. 1993. Vitamin E consumption and the risk of coronary disease in women. *New England Journal of Medicine* 328 (20):1444–49.

Stephens, N. G., A. Parsons, P. M. Schofield, F. Kelly, K. Cheeseman, and M. J. Mitchinson. 1996. Randomised controlled trial of vitamin E in patients with coronary disease: Cambridge Heart Antioxidant Study (CHAOS). *Lancet* 347 (9004):781–86.

Stump, D. D., and H. S. Gilbert. 1984. The effect of dietary vitamin E supplementation on a-tocopherol levels of human plasma and red blood cells. *Annals of the New York Academy of Sciences* 435:497–98.

Suzuki, Y. J., M. Tsuchiya, S. R. Wassall, Y. M. Choo, G. Govil, V. E. Kagan, and L. Packer. 1993. Structural and dynamic membrane properties of alpha-tocopherol and alpha-tocotrienol: implication to the molecular mechanism of their antioxidant potency. *Biochemistry* 32:10692–99.

Tan, B. 1992. Antitumor effects of palm carotenes and tocotrienols in HRS/J hairless female mice. *Nutrition Research* 12:S163–73.

Tappel, A. L. 1997. Vitamin E as a biological lipid antioxidant. *Inform* 8 (4):392–95.

Traber, M. G., and L. Packer. 1995. Vitamin E: Beyond antioxidant function. *American Journal of Clinical Nutrition* 62:S1501–09.

———, N. Podda, C. Weber, J. Thiele, M. Rallis, and L. Packer. 1997. Diet derived topically applied tocotrienols accumulate in skin and protect the tissue against UV light-induced oxidative stress. *Asia Pacific Journal of Clinical Nutrition* 6:63–67.

Watkins, T. R., P. Lenz, A. Gapor, M. Struck, A. Tomeo, and M. L. Bierenbaum. 1993. a-tocotrienol as a hypocholesterolemic and antioxidant agent in rats fed atherogenic diets. *Lipids* 28:1113–18.

Wechter, W. J., D. Kantoci, E. D. Murray, D. C. D'Amico, M. E. Jung, and W. H. Wang. 1996. A new endogenous natriuretic factor: LLU-a. *Proceedings of the National Academy of Sciences.* 93:6002–07.

6 Vitamin C: The Hub of the Network

Bendich, A., and L. Langseth. 1995. The health effects of vitamin C supplementation: A review. *Journal of the American College of Nutrition* 14:124–36.

Blanchard, J., T. N. Tozer, and M. Rowland. 1997. Pharmacokinetic perspectives on megadoses of ascorbic acid. *American Journal of Clinical Nutrition* 66 (5):1165–71.

Block, G. 1991. Vitamin C and cancer prevention: The epidemiologic evidence. *American Journal of Clinical Nutrition* 53 (suppl. 1):270–82.

Enstrom, J. E. 1997. Vitamin C in prospective epidemiological studies. *Vitamin C in Health and Disease,* edited by L. Packer and J. Fuchs. New York: Marcel Dekker.

Fraga, C. G., P. A. Motchnik, M. K. Shigenaga, H. J. Helbock, R. A. Jacob, and B. N. Ames. 1991. Ascorbic acid protects against endogenous oxidative DNA damage in human sperm. *Proceedings of the National Academy of Sciences* 88 (24):11003–06.

Gershoff, S. N. 1993. Vitamin C (ascorbic acid): New roles, new requirements? *Nutrition Reviews* 51:313–26.

Johnston, C. S., C. G. Meyer, and J. C. Srilakshmi. 1993. Vitamin C elevates red blood cell glutathione in healthy adults. *American Journal of Clinical Nutrition* 58 (1):103–05.

Levine, M., C. Conry-Cantilena, Y. Wang, R. W. Welch, P. W. Washko, K. R. Dhariwal, J. B. Park, A. Lazarev, J. F. Graumlich, and J. King. 1996. Vitamin C pharmacokinetics in healthy volunteers: Evidence for a recommended dietary allowance. *Proceedings of the National Academy of Sciences* 93 (8):3704–09.

Pinnell, S. R., S. Murad, and D. Darr. 1987. Induction of collagen synthesis by ascorbic acid. *Archives of Dermatology* 123:1684–86.

Robertson, J. M., A. P. Donner, and J. R. Trevithick. 1991. A possible role for vitamins C and E in cataract prevention. *American Journal of Clinical Nutrition* 53 (suppl. 1):346–51.

Woodall, A. A., and B. N. Ames. 1997. Diet and oxidative damage to DNA: The importance of ascorbate as an antioxidant. *Vitamin C in Health and Disease*, edited by L. Packer and J. Fuchs. New York: Marcel Dekker.

7   Coenzyme Q10: The Heart-Healthy Antioxidant

Beal, M. F., D. R. Henshaw, B. G. Jenkins, B. R. Rosen, and J. B. Schulz. 1994. Coenzyme Q10 and nicotinamide block striatal lesions produced by the mitochondrial toxin malonate. *Annals of Neurology* 36 (6):882–88.

Ernster, L., and G. Dallner. 1995. Biochemical, physiological, and medical aspects of ubiquinone function. *Biochimica et Biophysica Acta* 1271:195–204.

Frei, B., M. C. Kim, and B. N. Ames. 1990. Ubiquinol-10 is an effective lipid-soluble antioxidant at physiological concentrations. *Proceedings of the National Academy of Sciences* 87:4879–83.

Hanioka, T., M. Tanaka, M. Ojima, S. Shizukuishi, and K. Folkers. 1994. Effect of topical application of coenzyme Q10 on adult periodontitis. *Molecular Aspects of Medicine* 15 (suppl.):241–48.

Kagan, V. E., E. A. Serbinova, and L. Packer. 1990. Antioxidant effects of ubiquinones in microsomes and mitochondria are mediated by tocopherol recycling. *Biochemical and Biophysical Research Communications* 169:851–57.

Koroshetz, W. J., B. G. Jenkins, B. R. Rosen, and M. F. Beal. 1997. Energy metabolism defects in Huntington's disease and effects of coenzyme Q10. *Annals of Neurology* 41 (2):160–65.

Langsjoen, P. H., K. Folkers, K. Lyson, K. Muratsu, T. Lyson, and P. Langsjoen. 1990. Pronounced increase of survival of patients with cardiomyopathy when treated with coenzyme Q10 and conventional therapy. *International Journal of Tissue Reactions* 12 (3):163–68.

Lass, A., S. Agawal, and R. S. Sohal. 1997. Mitochondrial ubiquinone honologues, superoxide radical generation, and longevity in different mammalian species. *Journal of Biological Chemistry* 272:19199–204.

Lockwood, K., S. Moesgaard, T. Hanioka, and K. Folkers. 1994. Apparent partial remission of breast cancer in "high risk" patients supplemented with nutritional antioxidants, essential fatty acids and coenzyme Q10. *Molecular Aspects of Medicine* 15 (suppl.):S231–40.

Mohr, D., V. W. Bowry, and R. Stocker. 1992. Dietary supplementation with coenzyme Q10 results in increased levels of ubiquinol-10 within circulating lipoproteins and increased resistance of human low-density lipoprotein to the initiation of lipid peroxidation. *Biochimica et Biophysica Acta* 1126:247–54.

Nakamura, R., G. P. Littarru, K. Folkers, and E. G. Wilkinson. 1974. Study of Co Q10 enzymes in gingiva from patients with periodontal disease and evidence for a deficiency of coenzyme Q10. *Proceedings of the National Academy of Sciences* 71 (4):1456–60.

8 Glutathione: Nature's Master Antioxidant

Brack, C., E. Bechter-Thüring, and M. Labuhn. 1997. N-acetylcysteine slows down aging and increases the life span of *Drosophila melanogaster*. *Cellular and Molecular Life Sciences* 53 (11–12):960–66.

Jones, D. P. 1995. Glutathione distribution in natural products: Absorption and tissue distribution. *Glutathione and Thioredoxin: Thiols in Signal Transduction and Gene Regulation*. In Vol. 252 of *Biothiols, Methods in Enzymology*, edited by L. Packer. San Diego: Academic Press.

Kalebic, T., A. Kinter, G. Poli, M. E. Anderson, A. Meister, and A. S. Fauci. 1991. Suppression of human immunodeficiency virus expression in chronically infected monocytic cells by glutathione, glutathione ester, and N-acetylcysteine. *Proceedings of the National Academy of Sciences* 88:986–90.

Meister, A. 1995. Glutathione metabolism. *Monothiols and Dithiols, Protein Thiols and Thiyl Radicals*. In Vol. 251 of *Biothiols, Methods in Enzymology*, edited by L. Packer. San Diego: Academic Press.

Richie, J. P. Jr., B. J. Mills, and C. A. Lang. 1987. Correction of a glutathione deficiency in the aging mosquito increases its longevity. *Proceedings of the Society for Experimental Biology and Medicine* 184 (1):113–17.

Wu, D., S. N. Meydani, J. Sastre, M. Hayek, and M. Meydani. 1994. In vitro glutathione supplementation enhances interleukin-2 production and mitogenic response of peripheral blood mononuclear cells from young and old subjects. *Journal of Nutrition* 124 (5):655–63.

9 The Flavonoids: The Healing Power of Plants

Cheshier, J. E., S. Ardestani-Kaboudanian, B. Liang, M. Araghiniknam, S. Chung, L. Lane, A. Castro, and R. R. Watson. 1996. Immunomodulation by Pycnogenol in retrovirus-infected or ethanol-fed mice. *Life Sciences* 58 (5):PL 87–96.

Drehsen, G. 1999. From ancient pine bark uses to Pycnogenol. In *Antioxidant Food Supplements in Human Health*, edited by L. Packer, T. Yoshikawa, and M. Hiramatsu. San Diego: Academic Press.

Haramaki, N., L. Packer, M. T. Droy-Lefaix, and T. Christen. 1996. Antioxidant actions and health implications of ginkgo biloba extract. *Handbook of Antioxidants*, edited by E. Cadenas and L. Packer. New York: Marcel Dekker.

———, S. Aggarwal, T. Kawabata, M. T. Droy-Lefaix, and L. Packer. 1994. Effects of natural antioxidant ginkgo biloba extract (EGb 761) on myocardial ischemia-reperfusion injury. *Free Radical Biology & Medicine* 16:789–94.

Hertog, M. G., E. J. Feskens, P. C. Hollman, M. B. Katan, and D. Kromhout. 1993. Dietary antioxidant flavonoids and risk of coronary heart disease: The Zutphen Elderly Study. *Lancet* 342 (8878):1007–11.

Keli, S. O., M. G. Hertog, E. J. Feskens, and D. Kromhout. 1996. Dietary flavonoids, antioxidant vitamins, and incidence of stroke: The Zutphen study. *Archives of Internal Medicine* 156 (6):637–42.

Kinsella, J. E., E. Frankel, B. German, and J. Kanner. 1993. Possible mechanisms for the protective role of antioxidants in wine and plant foods. *Food Technology* 47 (4):85–89.

Kleijnen, J., and P. Knipschild. 1992. Ginkgo biloba for cerebral insufficiency. *British Journal of Clinical Pharmacology* 34 (4):352–58.

Knekt, P., R. Jarvinen, A. Reunanen, and J. Maatela. 1996. Flavonoid intake and coronary mortality in Finland: A cohort study. *British Medical Journal* (Clinical Research Ed.) 312 (7029):478–81.

———, R. Jarvinen, R. Seppanen, M. Hellovaara, L. Teppo, E. Pukkala, and A. Aromaa. 1997. Dietary flavonoids and the risk of lung cancer and other malignant neoplasms. *American Journal of Epidemiology* 146 (3):223–30.

Le Bars, P. L., M. M. Katz, N. Berman, T. M. Itil, A. M. Freedman, and F. A. Schatzberg. 1997. A placebo-controlled, double-blind, randomized trial of an extract of ginkgo biloba for dementia. North American EGb Study Group. *Journal of the American Medical Association* 278 (16):1327–32.

Noda, Y., K. Anzai, A. Mori, M. Kohno, M. Shinmei, and L. Packer. 1997. Hydroxyl and superoxide anion radical scavenging activities of natural source antioxidants using the computerized JES-FR30 ESR spectrometer system. *Biochemistry and Molecular Biology International* 42:35–44.

Packer, L., C. Saliou, M. T. Droy-Lefaix, and Y. Christen. 1998. Ginkgo biloba extract EGb761: Biological actions, antioxidant activity, and regulation of nitric oxide synthase. In Vol. 7 of *Flavonoids in Health and Disease,* edited by C. Rice-Evans and L. Packer. New York: Marcel Dekker.

Rice-Evans, C. A., N. J. Miller, and G. Paganga. 1996. Structure-antioxidant activity relationships of flavonoids and phenolic acids. Published erratum appears in *Free Radical Biology & Medicine* 21 (3):417. *Free Radical Biology & Medicine* 20 (7):933–56.

Rohdewald, P. 1998. Pycnogenol. In Vol. 7 of *Flavonoids in Health and Disease,* edited by C. Rice-Evans and L. Packer. New York: Marcel Dekker.

Rong, Y., L. Li, V. Shah, and B. H. Lau. 1995. Pycnogenol protects vascular endothelial cells from t-butyl hydroperoxide-induced oxidant injury. *Biotechnology Therapeutics* 5 (3–4):117–26.

Soleas, G. J., E. P. Diamandis, and D. M. Goldberg. 1997. Wine as a biological fluid: History, production, and role in disease prevention. *Journal of Clinical Laboratory Analysis* 11 (5):287–313.

Virgili, F., H. Kobuchi, Y. Noda, E. Cossins, and L. Packer. 1999. Pro-cyanidins from *Pinus maritima* bark: Antioxidant activity, effects on the immune system and modulation of nitrogen monoxide metabolism. In *Antioxidant Food Supplements in Human Health,* edited by L. Packer, T. Yoshikawa, and M. Hiramatsu. San Diego: Academic Press.

———, H. Kobuchi, and L. Packer. 1998. Nitrogen monoxide (NO) metabolism: Antioxidant properties and modulation of inducible NO synthase activity in activated macrophages by procyanidins extracted from *Pinus maritima* (Pycnogenol). *Flavonoids in Health and Disease,* edited by C. Rice-Evans and L. Packer. New York: Marcel Dekker.

10 The Controversial Carotenoids

The Alpha-Tocopherol, Beta Carotene Cancer Prevention Study Group. 1994. The effect of vitamin E and beta carotene on the incidence of lung cancer and other cancers in male smokers. *New England Journal of Medicine* 330 (15):1029–35.

Blot, W. J., J. Y. Li, P. R. Taylor, W. Guo, S. Dawsey, G. Q. Wang, C. S. Yang, S. F. Zheng, M. Gail, G. Y. Li, Y. Yu, B. Liu, J. Tangrea, Y. Sun, F. Liu, J. F. Fraumeni, Y. H. Zhang, and B. Li. 1993. Nutrition intervention trials in Linxian, China: Supplementation with specific vitamin/mineral combinations, cancer incidence, and disease-specific mortality in the general population. *Journal of the National Cancer Institute* 85 (18):1483–92.

Clinton, S. K. 1998. Lycopene: Chemistry, biology and implications for human health and disease. *Nutrition Reviews* 56 (2):35–51.

Giovannucci, E., and S. K. Clinton. 1998. Tomatoes, lycopene, and prostate cancer. Prostate Cancer. *Proceedings of the Society for Experimental Biology and Medicine* 218 (2):129–39.

Krinsky, N. I. 1993. Actions of carotenoids in biological systems. *Annual Review of Nutrition* 13:561–87.

Mayne, S. T. 1996. Beta-carotene, carotenoids and disease prevention in humans. *The Federation of American Societies for Experimental Biology (FASEB) Journal,* 10:690–701.

Omenn, G. S., G. E. Goodman, M. D. Thornquist, J. Balmes, M. R. Cullen, A. Glass, J. P. Keogh, F. L. Meyskens Jr., B. Valanis, J. H. Williams Jr., et al. 1996. Risk factors for lung cancer and for intervention effects in CARET, the Beta-Carotene and Retinol Efficacy Trial. *Journal of the National Cancer Institute* 88 (21):1550–59.

Rock, C. L. 1997. Carotenoids: Biology and treatment. *Pharmacology and Therapeutics* 75:185–97.

Sies, H., and W. Stahl. 1995. Vitamins E and C, beta-carotene and other carotenoids as antioxidants. *American Journal of Clinical Nutrition* 62:1315S–21S.

11 The Selenium Surprise

Blot, W. J., J. Y. Li, P. R. Taylor, W. Guo, S. Dawsey, G. Q. Wang, C. S. Yang, S. F. Zheng, M. Gail, G. Y. Li, Y. Yu, B. Liu, J. Tangrea, Y. Sun, F. Liu, J. F. Fraumeni, Y. H. Zhang, and B. Li. 1993. Nutrition intervention trials in Linxian, China: Supplementation with specific vitamin/mineral combinations, cancer incidence, and disease-specific mortality in the general population. *Journal of the National Cancer Institute* 85 (18):1483–92.

Clark, L. C., B. Dalkin, A. Krongrad, G. F. Combs Jr., B. W. Turnbull, E. H. Slate, R. Witherington, J. H. Herlong, E. Janosko, D. Carpenter, C. Borosso, S. Falk, and J. Rounder. 1998. Decreased incidence of prostate cancer with selenium supplementation: Result of a double-blind cancer prevention trial. *British Journal of Urology* 81 (5):730–34.

————, G. F. Combs Jr., B. W. Turnbull, E. H. Slate, D. K. Chalker, J. Chow, L. S. Davis, R. A. Glover, G. F. Graham, E. G. Gross, A. Krongrad, J. L. Lesher, H. K. Park, B. B. Sanders, C. L. Smith, and R. Taylor. 1996. Effects of selenium supplementation for cancer prevention in patients with carcinoma of the skin. A randomized controlled trial. Nutritional Prevention of Cancer Study Group. *Journal of the American Medical Association* 276 (24):1957–63.

Garland, M., M. J. Stampfer, W. C. Willett, and D. J. Hunter. 1994. The epidemiology of selenium and human cancer. In *Natural Antioxidants in Human Health and Disease,* edited by B. Frei. New York: Academic Press.

Kardinaal, A. F., F. J. Kok, L. Kohlmeier, J. M. Martin-Moreno, J. Ringstad, J. Gomez-Aracena, V. P. Mazaev, M. Thamm, B. C. Martin, A. Aro, et al. 1997. Association between toenail selenium and risk of acute myocardial infarction in European men. The EURAMIC Study. European Antioxidant Myocardial Infarction and Breast Cancer. *American Journal of Epidemiology* 145 (4):373–79.

Knekt, P., J. Marniemi, L. Teppo, M. Heliövaara, and A. Aromaa. 1998. Is low selenium a risk factor of lung cancer? *American Journal of Epidemiology* 148 (no. 10).

Salvini, S., C. H. Hennekens, J. S. Morris, W. C. Willett, and M. J. Stampfer. 1995. Plasma levels of the antioxidant selenium and risk of myocardial infarction among U.S. physicians. *American Journal of Cardiology* 76 (17):1218–21.

van den Brandt, P. A., R. A. Goldbohm, P. van 't Veer, P. Bode, E. Dorant, R. J. Hermus, and F. Sturmans. 1993. A prospective cohort study on selenium status and the risk of lung cancer. *Cancer Research* 53 (20):4860–65.

van Poppel, G., A. Kardinaal, H. Princen, and F. J. Kok. 1994. Antioxidants and coronary heart disease. *Annals of Medicine* 26 (6):429–34.

Virtamo, J., and J. K. Huttunen. 1998. Minerals, trace elements and cardiovascular disease. An overview. *Annals of Clinical Research* 20 (1–2):102–13.

12 Fulfilling the Antioxidant Miracle: Achieving Optimal Health

Aruoma, O. I. 1994. Nutrition and health aspects of free radicals and antioxidants. *Food and Chemical Toxicology* 32:671–83.

Halliwell, B. 1994. Free radicals and antioxidants: A personal view. *Nutrition Reviews* 53:253–65.

Jacob, R. A. 1995. The integrated antioxidant system. *Nutrition Research* 15 (5):755–76.

Packer, L., and J. L. Sullivan. 1995. The promise of antioxidants. *The Saturday Evening Post* (January/February).

13 An Antioxidant Feast: Food Is Powerful Medicine

Block, G., B. Patterson, and A. Subar. 1992. Fruit, vegetables, and cancer prevention: A review of the epidemiological evidence. *Nutrition and Cancer* 18 (1):1–29.

Caragay, A. B. 1992. Cancer-preventive foods and ingredients. *Food Technology* 65–68.

Hara, Y. 1997. Prophylactic functions of antioxidant tea polyphenols. In *Food Factors for Chemistry and Cancer Prevention,* edited by H. Ohigashi, T. Osawa, J. Terao, S. Watanabe, and T. Yoshikawa. Tokyo: Springer-Verlag.

Jacobs, M. M. 1993. Diet, nutrition, and cancer research: An overview. *Nutrition Today* 28 (3):19–23.

Korver, O. 1997. Tea components and cancer prevention. In *Food Factors for Chemistry and Cancer Prevention,* edited by H. Ohigashi, T. Osawa, J. Terao, S. Watanabe, and T. Yoshikawa. Tokyo: Springer-Verlag.

Lee, H. P., L. Gourley, S. W. Duffy, J. Esteve, J. Lee, and N. E. Day. 1991. Dietary effects on breast-cancer risk in Singapore. *Lancet* 337 (8751):1197–200.

Phelps, S., and W. S. Harris. 1993. Garlic supplementation and lipoprotein oxidation susceptibility. *Lipids* 28 (5):475–77.

Weisburger, J. H. 1997. Dietary fat and risk of chronic disease: Mechanistic insights from experimental studies. *Journal of the American Dietetic Association* 97 (suppl. 7):16–23.

Yang, C. S., and Z. Y. Wang. 1993. Tea and cancer. *Journal of the National Cancer Institute* 85 (13):1038–49.

Ziegler, R. G. 1991. Vegetables, fruits, and carotenoids and the risk of cancer. *American Journal of Clinical Nutrition* 53 (suppl. 1):251–59.

14 The Packer Plan: Your Supplement Regimen

Gey, F. K. 1995. Ten-year retrospective on the antioxidant hypothesis of arteriosclerosis: Threshold plasma levels of antioxidant micronutrients related to minimum cardiovascular risk. *Nutritional Biochemistry* 6:206–36.

Tribble, D. L., L. J. Giuliano, and S. P. Fortmann. 1993. Reduced plasma ascorbic acid concentrations in nonsmokers regularly exposed to environmental tobacco smoke. *American Journal of Clinical Nutrition* 58 (6):886–90.

15 The Packer Plan: Antioxidants for Healthy, Beautiful Skin

Darr, D. J., R. M. Colven, and S. R. Pinnell. 1997. Topical vitamin C. *Vitamin C in Health and Disease,* edited by L. Packer and J. Fuchs. New York: Marcel Dekker.

Darr, D., S. Combs, S. Dunston, T. Manning, and S. Pinnell. 1992. Topical vitamin C protects porcine skin from ultraviolet radiation-induced damage. *British Journal of Dermatology* 127 (3):247–53.

Fuchs, F., and L. Packer. 1993. Vitamin E in dermatological therapy. *Vitamin E in Health and Disease,* edited by J. Fuchs and L. Packer. New York: Marcel Dekker.

Fuchs, J., M. E. Huflejt, L. M. Rothfuss, D. S. Wilson, G. Carcamo, and L. Packer. 1989. Acute effects of near ultraviolet and visible light on the cutaneous antioxidant defense system. *Photochemistry and Photobiology* 50:739–44.

Lopez-Torres, M., J. J. Thiele, Y. Shindo, D. Han, and L. Packer. 1998. Topical application of a-tocopherol modulates the antioxidant network and diminishes ultraviolet-induced oxidative damage in murine skin. *British Journal of Dermatology* 138:207–15.

Phillips, C. L., S. B. Combs, and S. R. Pinnell. 1994. Effects of ascorbic acid on proliferation and collagen synthesis in relation to the donor age of human dermal fibroblasts. *Journal of Investigative Dermatology* 103 (2):228–32.

Shindo, Y., E. Witt, D. Han, and L. Packer. 1994. Dose-response effects of acute ultraviolet irradiation on antioxidants and molecular markers of oxidation in murine epidermis and dermis. *Journal of Investigative Dermatology* 102:470–75.

Thiele, J., M. Podda, and L. Packer. 1997. Tropospheric ozone: An emerging environmental stress to skin. *Biological Chemistry* 378:1299–305.

———, M. G. Traber, and L. Packer. 1998. Depletion of human stratum corneum vitamin E: An early and sensitive in vivo marker of UV-induced photo-oxidation. *Journal of Investigative Dermatology* 110:756–61.

———, M. Podda, et al. 1997. Ozone depletes tocopherols and tocotrienols topically applied to murine skin. *The Federation of European Biochemical Societies (FEBS) Letters* 401:167–70.

———, et al. 1997. In vivo exposure to ozone depletes vitamins C and E and induces lipid peroxidation in epidermal layers of murine skin. *Free Radical Biology & Medicine* 23:385–91.

Traber, M., M. Rallis, M. Podda, C. Weber, H. Maibach, and L. Packer. 1998. Penetration and distribution of alpha-tocopherol, alpha- or gamma-tocotrienols applied individually onto murine skin. *Lipids* 33:87–91.

Weber, C., M. Podda, M. Rallis, J. J. Thiele, M. G. Traber, and L. Packer. 1997. Efficacy of topically applied tocopherols and tocotrienols in protection of murine skin from oxidative damage induced by UV-irradiation. *Free Radical Biology & Medicine* 22:761–69.

CPSIA information can be obtained at www.ICGtesting.com
Printed in the USA
BVOW05*1820210914

367742BV00004B/12/P